Six Roads To Glory
by Cawood Ledford

Host Communications, Inc.
Lexington, Kentucky

"Six Roads To Glory" is published by Host Communications, Inc., 904 North Broadway, Lexington, Kentucky 40505. W. James Host, Publisher; Richard A. Ford, President; Eric Barnhart, Vice President

Photography by Brian Spurlock, Rich Clarkson, Bill Straus, Brooks Downing. Additional photos provided by the University of Kentucky Media Relations Office, the University of Kentucky Special Collections and Ralph Beard

Project Manager: Kim Ramsay
Promotions and Distribution: Laura Mize
Edited by David Kaplan
Cover artwork by Michael J. Taylor
Editorial assistance by Dave Mrvos, Craig Baroncelli, Jai Giffin, Jim Kelsey, Pat Henderson, Dan Peters, Mark Buerger, Pete Rhoda, Ashley Beavers, Steve Downey, Beth Whitmore, Dan Hargett, Samantha Skaggs, Lori Holladay, Steve Kirkwood, Jennifer Johnson, Jennifer Miller, Kristin Emerling
Design by Jamie Barker and Jeff Quire
Design assistance by Dana Bart, Joe Miller, Tara Yurkshat

ISBN: 1-57640-023-9

Six Roads To Glory
by Cawood Ledford

To dear friends

Jim and Pat Host
C.M. and Evelyn Newton
Rick and Joanne Pitino

Acknowledgements

Writing a book about Kentucky basketball is a labor of love but it takes the cooperation of several people to get it done. At least it did for this one.

My thanks to Jim Host, who conceived the idea for this book and offered his encouragement all the way through. My gratitude to Kim Ramsay, who nourished the manuscript from beginning to end and to my wife, Frances, for her proofing and editing skills.

I couldn't have written this book without the cooperation of the former players who gave unselfishly of their time and knowledge.

For the 1940s, many thanks to Wallace "Wah Wah" Jones and Humzey Yessin and a special thanks to Ralph Beard, who not only was very helpful in his contributions, but who also made his private photos available to us.

For the 1950s, Frank Ramsey and Bobby Watson were very generous with their help.

For the 1970s, a special thanks to Joe B. Hall, who coached the great 1978 team and recalled that season for us.

For the 1990s, Rick Pitino couldn't have been more giving of his time and knowledge.

Foreword

Winning championships is what it's all about. It's the standard by which greatness in sports is judged, whether it's a team sport like basketball or an individual sport like tennis or golf. Few people ever remember the runner-up. However, hoist the championship trophy and your name is forever etched in our memory and in the history books.

The mark of true greatness lies in consistency. Teams or individuals that perform at a championship level, year in and year out, are the ones that are most impressive, the ones who deserve our deepest admiration. Many teams and players sneak up, have a good year, win a title, then revert back to mediocrity. That's the rule rather than the exception. For whatever reason — or reasons — they don't have the ability, discipline or strength of character to keep their grip on the mountain top.

Of course, it's not easy getting to the top, and it's even more difficult staying there once you do. When you're the king, everyone wants your crown. Slip up for a second, let your guard down just a bit, or ease off on your work ethic and the crown that you once wore so proudly now sits on the head of someone else.

That's why it's impossible not to appreciate the Chicago Bulls for what they've accomplished. The same goes for the old Boston

Celtics and the New York Yankees. Even if they weren't your favorite teams, you can't help but be impressed by what they accomplished over so many years. I don't care what sport you're talking about. To win all those championships and to consistently maintain such a high level of excellence is deserving of our respect and admiration.

Without question, I think the same holds true for the University of Kentucky basketball program. Many programs have risen to the top, had their moment in the sun, then fallen on hard times. Many other programs have been excellent for the past 25, 30 or 35 years. But can you name another college basketball program that comes close to matching Kentucky's level of sustained excellence over such a long period of time? I can't. Think about it. Kentucky has been one of the premier basketball programs for seven decades, going back to the early 1930s, when Adolph Rupp took over as head coach. Down through those years, Kentucky has set the standard that others have struggled mightily to achieve and maintain.

When we won the national title in 1996, it marked the sixth time the school has hoisted a championship banner. Six titles under three different coaches — I think that says a lot about the strength and consistency of the Kentucky basketball program.

No one knows more about the rich tradition of University of Kentucky basketball than Cawood Ledford. After all, for 39 winters Cawood was an integral part of that tradition, the name whose unmistakable voice brought the action on the court into the living rooms of thousands of loyal Big Blue fans. His words painted the pictures long before the Wildcats were on television. It was Cawood who linked the fans to their hardwood heroes.

In his book, "Six Roads To Glory," Cawood gives us a close-up look at each of Kentucky's six national championship teams. He begins with the 1996 club, the one that I had the good fortune to coach, then shifts back to the beginning of the Glory Days with the fabled Fabulous Five team that won the school's first national title in 1948. Then comes Rupp-coached championship teams in 1949, 1951 and 1958, followed by Joe B. Hall's tough 1978 team that won it all in St. Louis.

Cawood reflects on the big moments in key games, the coaches and the players who made it happen. The list of stars who led UK's championship teams is nothing less than a "Who's Who" of Wildcat greats — Ralph Beard, Alex Groza, Bill Spivey, Cliff Hagan, Frank Ramsey, Johnny Cox, Vernon Hatton, Kyle Macy, Jack Givens, Tony Delk, Antoine Walker. Outstanding players who performed at the top of their game when it counted the most.

In addition, Cawood dedicates a chapter to the 1953-54 team, the one led by future Basketball Hall of Fame players Hagan and Ramsey, that sailed through the season with an unblemished 25-0 record, only to turn down the opportunity to participate in the NCAA Tournament. Cawood tells us how that strange turn of events came about, and why he's convinced that that club would have won it all had it participated.

He closes the book with a chapter on the 1996-97 club, a team that surprised everyone — including me — by making it all the way to the championship game before losing in overtime to Arizona. Why would Cawood include this team? That's an easy one to answer. Cawood has a tremendous appreciation for players and teams that display the ultimate in courage, heart and tenacity. He loves overachievers, and believe me, this year's team certainly fits that category.

This book is a most enjoyable ride down what has been a road lined with basketball riches. It is a continuing story, one filled with heroic performances from a host of Wildcat players, young men whose will, desire and strength of character elevated the University of Kentucky to the pinnacle of the college basketball world.

Once again, as only he can do, Cawood Ledford has given new life to our glorious past.

Rick Pitino

Rick Pitino

It Could Have Been Box-Ball

If the YMCA janitor had been more resourceful, we might be playing the game of basketball with square hoops today.

Faced with the necessity of developing a sport that could be played indoors during the New England winter of 1891, Dr. James Naismith's fertile mind conjured up a game to be played with a soccer ball. Running and tackling would not be allowed and the only way to score was to put the ball in a goal at the end of the gym.

The good doctor asked the janitor to find him two wooden boxes about 18 inches square. Instead of searching for the boxes, the custodian came up with two peach baskets he had on hand and we have basketball instead of box-ball.

The game of basketball was born in Springfield, Massachusetts, sometime in December 1891. The game was an instant hit, first gaining wide popularity among the YMCAs across the country. Not long after, the colleges embraced the game.

The college game received its first national exposure when Ned Irish, a former newspaper man, began promoting a doubleheader each year in what was in those days the Mecca of the game, Madison Square Garden. He would invite a pair of well-known teams from around the country to play against two teams from the New York area. It was an immediate success.

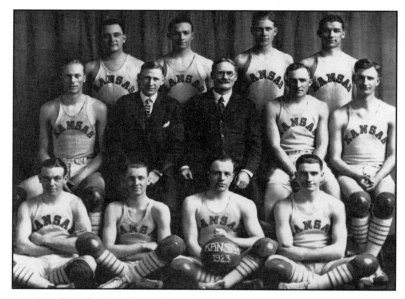

During his playing days at Kansas, Adolph Rupp (top, left) was influenced by the founder of basketball, Dr. James Naismith (third, middle row).

Irish outdid himself in 1938 when he devised the first National Invitation Tournament to be held at the Garden. It began with six teams, and again, was a great success both artistically and financially.

The nation's coaches admired the accomplishments of Irish but they wanted to get in on the action. At the National Basketball Coaches Association convention the next April, they decided to have their own tournament. The coaches went to the NCAA to get their plans approved. The NCAA sanctioned the tournament but wanted the coaches to run the show.

The first tournament was set for 1939 with the coaches picking a team from each of eight regions of the country. Four teams would play in the West and the other four in the East with the two winners meeting at a different site for the championship. Oregon won the first NCAA Tournament with a 46-33 win over Ohio State, in Evanston, Illinois. The operation was a success but the patient died.

For all tournament games, fewer than 16,000 bought tickets and the tournament lost more than $2,500. The coaches proved better at coaching than they did at administrating. They went back to the NCAA and convinced that organization to take over the tournament the next year. Since then, everything has been coming up roses. Each year it just seems to get bigger and bigger and better and better, and now the Final Four ranks among the top sports classics held each year in this country.

The NCAA Tournament is really something special. The only way it can be won is in the arena. Football championships are determined by polls, sportswriters or coaches ... but to win basketball's big trophy, the teams have to undergo the test of survival. When the smoke clears, only one team is left undefeated in the big postseason classic.

For my money, the two things that have been most responsible for the tremendous success of the NCAA Tournament have been (1) the expansion of the number of teams invited; and (2) moving teams to different regions in order to strengthen those regions.

For the 1939 inaugural tournament, a coach was put in charge of inviting a team from his region. That was the way the eight teams were chosen. As time went by, there were more then a few complaints that some coaches were choosing their cronies and some deserving teams were left at home. Kentucky's Adolph Rupp always thought politics cost his 1950 team a trip to the "big show." The Cats were the defending NCAA champions and returned that season with a 25-4 record, winning their last 14 games in a row. It's doubtful that Kentucky would have won the NCAA because the Cats went to the NIT and were blasted 89-50 by City College of New York. CCNY won the NCAA Championship 10 days later.

In 1951, the tournament field was doubled to 16 teams with 10 conference champions qualifying automatically. The Southeastern Conference was among them.

By 1975, the number of bids had grown to 32 and for the first time, more than one team from the same conference could go to the NCAA Tournament. The very next year, Indiana and Michigan, both from the Big Ten, met for the title. Indiana won, 86-68.

In 1985, the tournament field was expanded to its present 64 teams. There has been talk of letting all Division I teams participate in the postseason classic but, in my opinion, this would weaken the tournament. They just about have it perfect with the best 64 teams taking part.

The NCAA Basketball Committee does an incredible job of choosing the teams, then seeding them and placing those teams into the four regions. Oh, there are always some complaints from teams that don't make it or about the order of the seeding for those that do but, for the most part, things go smoothly.

All the Division I college teams dream of making the NCAA Tournament field and it is a great honor to be chosen. No guarantees go with the invitation. Facing the best teams in the country, game after game, is a tough row to hoe. To win the national championship is one of the most difficult tasks in sports. To win six straight games against the caliber of competition is no walk in the park.

To begin with, the best team doesn't always win the championship. Not by a long shot. It's one and done. It would be a better measure of the best team if they did what the pros do, play a best of seven series. Still, there is that extra excitement in single elimination. Coach Rupp was heard to grumble at the beginning of any tournament, "There's no tomorrow."

To win the "big dance," a team has to have several ingredients. First, and perhaps most important, it must have talent. None of the lower seeds have ever won. They just don't have the manpower to make it all the way.

The winner must have depth. When Kentucky lost that heartbreaker to Duke in 1992 in the final two seconds of overtime in the Elite Eight, Gimel Martinez and Jamal Mashburn, UK's two tallest players, had already fouled out. When the Wildcats lost the next year to Michigan, in overtime at the Final Four, Mashburn again was on the bench with five fouls.

A winning NCAA Tournament team must be versatile. It has to be able to adjust to about any style of play. The great teams can play at any tempo.

A national championship team ALWAYS plays great defense. When the shots aren't going in, a superb defense will save that team. The 1996 Wildcat team is a perfect example. After a gut-wrenching win against Massachusetts, a weary Kentucky team had to come back two nights later to play Syracuse in the final. The Cats couldn't throw it against the side of a barn but their defense was so outstanding they were able to win anyway.

To win it all, a team must win the close games. Kentucky didn't have a game in 1996 that went right to the wire, where the last shot won. But it's hardly a blowout when a team leads by three (73-70), as Kentucky did against UMass with 1:02 remaining in the semifinal or by a two-point advantage (64-62) against Syracuse in the championship game, with less than five minutes to play.

The winning team must have luck. No, not just luck ... good luck. Here and there the last shot has to go in. It has to be lucky enough to avoid injuries at critical times. I still believe Kentucky would have beaten Michigan in the 1993 Final Four had Dale Brown not been forced to leave the game with an injury. Dale was having one of his best games.

Winning the NCAA Tournament is the highest honor that can come to a college basketball team. It's the top of the mountain. Kentucky has enjoyed reaching that pinnacle six times.

From the Pope to the President

From late summer of 1995 to early spring 1996, few teams have enjoyed the high exhilaration enjoyed by the Kentucky Wildcats. It all started when Rick Pitino took his team to Italy in August. This resulted in Rick and Joanne having an audience with Pope John Paul II. The marvelous journey ended April 1, 1996, when Pitino led the Wildcats to Kentucky's sixth NCAA Championship. Immediately after the victory over Syracuse in the final game at the Meadowlands Sports complex in East Rutherford, New Jersey, President Bill Clinton called to offer his congratulations and at the end of the spring semester, Clinton hosted Pitino and the Wildcats at the White House. It just doesn't get much better than that.

To understand just what a remarkable journey it had been for Pitino during his seven years at Kentucky, we must turn back the calendar to 1989, when he came on the scene. Kentucky was suffering through its darkest hour as a basketball program. The Cats were coming off their first losing season in 62 years. The NCAA had dealt the program some of the harshest penalties handed down in years ... no postseason play for two years ... no TV for one season ... two players were ruled ineligible to play at Kentucky and two others elected to transfer. Under the NCAA penalty, no scholarships were available to replace them.

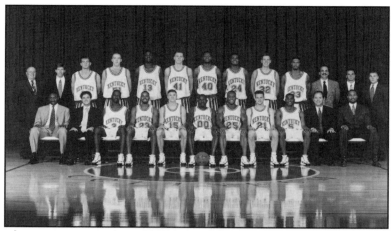

The 1995-96 Kentucky Wildcats. Front Row (L-R): Asst. Coach Delray Brooks, Head Coach Rick Pitino, Allen Edwards, Derek Anderson, Jeff Sheppard, Tony Delk, Anthony Epps, Cameron Mills, Wayne Turner, Assoc. Coach Jim O'Brien, Asst. Coach Winston Bennett. Back Row: Equip. Mgr. Bill Keightley, Admin. Asst. George Barber, Jason Lathrem, Oliver Simmons, Nazr Mohammed, Mark Pope, Walter McCarty, Antoine Walker, Jared Prickett, Ron Mercer, Trainer Eddie Jamiel, Asst. Strength Coach Layne Kaufman, Strength Coach Shaun Brown.

Pitino had only eight scholarship players on hand and none was taller than 6-7. Reggie Hanson and Derrick Miller had been starters on a losing team the previous season, but the other six had been bench warmers. In about as close to a miracle as you can get, Pitino led that rag-tag bunch to a 14-14 season.

The next year, the Cats had the best record in the SEC, but the penalties were still in place and there would be no postseason action for Kentucky.

For the 1991-92 season, the Cats had served their sentence and were ready to compete on equal terms with the other college teams. They won the SEC Tournament and went all the way to the NCAA Tournament's Elite Eight, before losing to the defending national champion Duke Blue Devils by one point in overtime.

The 1993 Wildcats won the SEC Tournament for the second year in a row and advanced to the Final Four before they were eliminated by Michigan in overtime.

The following season saw the Cats win the SEC Tournament for the third year in a row. They were eliminated in the second round of the NCAA Tournament by Marquette.

The 1995 team made it four in a row for Pitino by winning the SEC Tournament again. Rick had perhaps his best team that season and the Cats swept through the first and second round games of the NCAA Tournament in Memphis, over Mount St. Mary's and Tulane. They were favored to win the Southeast Regional in Birmingham, Alabama. Kentucky coasted by Arizona State, but the Cats were upset one game short of the Final Four by North Carolina, 74-61. That game still sticks in Pitino's craw.

"We were up in that game something like 10-2, when the referee called a double technical foul, which I thought was inappropriate," Pitino said. He gave a technical foul to Walter McCarty, who wasn't even in the play. Andre Riddick had his hands around Rasheed Wallace's neck after Wallace flagrantly threw him an elbow. Without question, both players probably deserved to be ejected. They weren't. Since a technical foul also counts as a personal foul, and Walter was called for another quick foul, I had to take him out of the game. We lost our momentum and we were all upset."

Pitino tried to get the official to reconsider the technical on McCarty, believing that if the official would check the video tape he would see that Walter wasn't even involved in the skirmish. Rick said the official, Tim Higgins, made a snide remark that Pitino should watch the tape that night on the news.

Despite the officiating, Pitino admits his team did not play well against North Carolina.

"We played a terrible basketball game," he said. "We did not play as a team. We came to the conclusion that we were never going to play that way again in the NCAA Tournament. That was our rallying cry for that spring, summer and the following year."

One of the most enjoyable times of my life was in 1995, when Frances and I accompanied the Wildcats on their tour of Italy. Rick invited us to go along, and it's a trip I'll remember to my dying day.

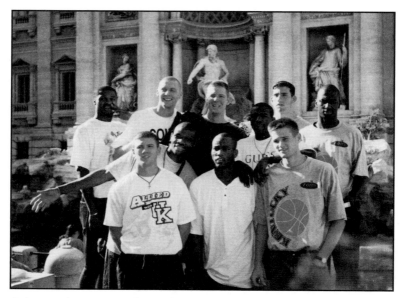

Prior to the season, the Wildcats visited Italy for a five-game exhibition tour.

We landed in Milan on the morning of August 13, and spent our first night at one of the leading hotels in the world, the Grand Hotel Villa D'Este, right on the banks of beautiful Lake Como. We traveled from there to UK's first game which produced an overtime win over Cagiva Varese. That same team was scheduled to play UK back in Lexington in one of the preseason exhibition games.

Venice was the next destination for the traveling party that included 10 players: Tony Delk, Allen Edwards, Anthony Epps, Walter McCarty, Cameron Mills, Scott Padgett, Jared Prickett, Mark Pope, Jeff Sheppard and Antoine Walker. On the way to Venice, we stopped off in Verona to look at the balcony that inspired Shakespeare to write "Romeo and Juliet." There was a statue in the courtyard of a young maiden and somehow a tradition had started that rubbing her left breast would bring good luck. As you would guess, cameras recorded that many in our traveling party took advantage to make sure Lady Luck was on their side, at least for the remainder of the trip. In Venice, I believe everybody took advantage of a gondola ride on the canal and watched the Wildcats defeat a local pro team and a touring team from Russia.

We moved on to Florence where the Cats lost for the only time in Italy, 123-115, at the hands of Montecatini. Even though Rick had insisted that it didn't really matter whether his team won or lost on the tour, when a pair of local officials made some ridiculous calls, his competitive juices kicked in and he picked up two technical fouls and was booted from the gym. Even though Rick is of Italian descent, he doesn't speak the language. He enlisted the help of one of the tour directors Roger Valdiserri, the former sports information director at Notre Dame, to sit with him on the bench and act as an interpreter. Rick didn't need Roger's help to get evicted. I sat right behind the bench and the insult he flung at the official might have been in English, but I believe it could have been understood in any language.

From Florence, the Wildcats traveled to their final destination, Rome. I enjoyed all the cities we visited, but I enjoyed Rome the most. We visited the Trevi Fountain, the centerpiece for the movie, "Three Coins in the Fountain." I think the players enjoyed touring the Colosseum the most, an ancient structure that seated 50,000 spectators when it was completed in 80 A.D. There had been a 100-day festival, we were told, that saw 9,000 wild beasts killed and 2,000 gladiators lose their lives.

A visit to Vatican City was really special with all of its art and statues on display. We were all really proud, watching Rick and Joanne go up to the stage to meet with the Pope.

"The thrill of a lifetime was getting an audience with the Pope for Joanne and myself," Rick told me. "Meeting the Pope was not something we envisioned would happen in our lifetimes. It was really quite special."

Back in this country, one of Pitino's favorite banquet jokes was that after he kissed the Pope's ring, the Pontiff offered to return the favor but alas, there was no Pitino ring. He had to delete that little joke after the 1996 team earned him one.

In Italy, Rick elected to just play the games and skip the practice sessions so that the players would be able to tour and participate in a wonderful and educational experience. The rules did not allow Pitino to take the freshmen nor Derek Anderson, who had sat out the previous season after transferring from Ohio State. Rick could only take the players who had played during the past season. Padgett went along although he would be ineligible until he straightened himself out academically. Rick thought the trip would do more than just improve the Cats' level of play.

"More than anything else, we bonded as a team," he said. "We really got to know each other. We got close. We had not been a close team from top to bottom but that trip really gave the players a chance to develop a strong, close relationship."

Remembering the North Carolina debacle that ended the Cats' 1995 run in the NCAA Tournament and brought their season to an abrupt and disappointing end, Pitino preached unselfishness from the first day of practice. He asked that every player sacrifice himself for the good of the team. He wanted them to think pass before shot. He wanted them to think of their teammates before themselves. He told them if they would do these things and develop an awesome defense, they would have a great opportunity to win the national championship. Pitino told his players, "If the team wins, you win. Your own agenda will be filled if you sacrifice yourself for the good of the team."

When the first preseason poll was announced, Kentucky was ranked No. 1. Pitino welcomed the ranking and the intense pressure it brought to the team.

"I told the players every week that they were the luckiest people in America because we had all this pressure on us. Pressure can be our best ally if we practice every practice as if a national championship was at stake." Turns out, it was.

All the players who made the trip to Italy were available for duty except Padgett, who would have to drop out of UK until he

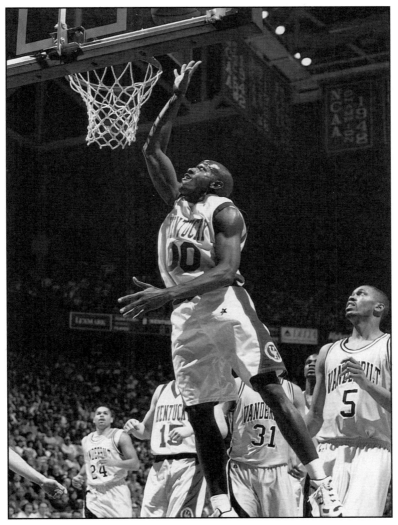

A shooting guard his first three seasons at UK, Tony Delk began the 1995-96 season as Kentucky's playmaker.

got his grades in better order. Joining the team would be Anderson, Ron Mercer, Wayne Turner and Nazr Mohammed. Gone from the previous season's squad were Andre Riddick and Chris Harrison who had played out their eligibility. Rodrick Rhodes had transferred to Southern Cal.

One night in Rome, Rick and I shared a cab on our way to having dinner with the head of the Italian Olympic Committee. Rick wondered what I thought of his moving Delk to point guard for the upcoming season. He had tried that before but always moved Tony back to the two-guard position, and I wondered whether his experiment would work. To enhance Delk's chances at a pro career, Pitino was adamant about giving the senior his shot at the point guard position. When the Wildcats opened the season against Maryland in the Tip-Off Classic, Tony opened at the point.

Delk was 6-1 but performed like a much taller player. He had long arms and could really jump. Tony had a tendency to be a streaky shooter from the perimeter but, when he had his stroke, he could destroy an opponent from long range.

Starting that opening game at the two-guard was Derek Anderson. Derek had a full season of practice after transferring from Ohio State and he had shown Pitino that he was an incredible player with his great quickness on both offense and defense. Rick had great success at Kentucky with transfers. He likes the maturity they bring and the full season he gets with them to learn the system before they begin play. Anderson had two years of eligibility remaining with the Wildcats.

Mark Pope started at center. Pope had also been a transfer, from Washington, but had become eligible at UK for the 1994-95 season and led the team in rebounding. The 6-10, 235-pound center was a hard-nosed player inside and could venture out to the perimeter and hit the three-pointer. Mark led the top-ranked Wildcats in their 1995-96 season-opening win over Maryland with 26 points as the Cats claimed the victory, 96-84.

In the Maryland game, Antoine Walker and freshman Ron Mercer opened at the forward positions. Walker, a 6-8 sophomore, had come to Kentucky with loads of offensive firepower but had to improve defensively. He was an intense competitor with a great desire to win. Antoine was a mentally tough player who was one of

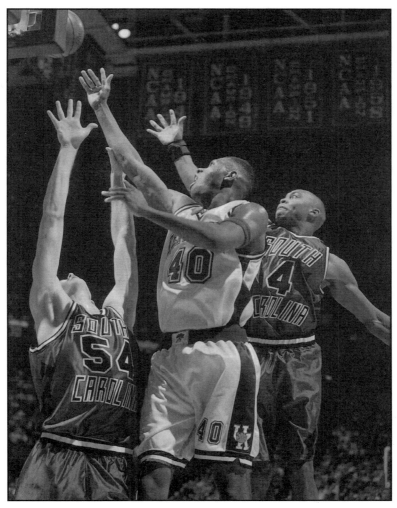

Walter McCarty possessed a well-rounded game that enabled him to score from the perimeter or on the blocks.

the best players Rick had brought to Kentucky.

Mercer was generally regarded as the best high school player in the country when Rick recruited the 6-7 star. There was no question of Mercer's talent. Few freshmen start the first game of the their career at Kentucky. Ron would start a dozen games for the Wild-

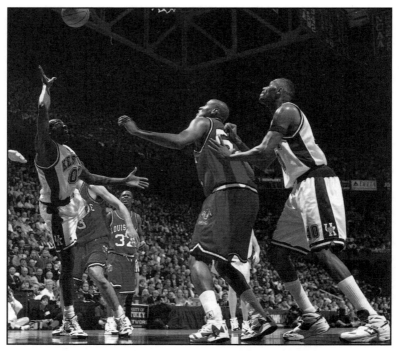

Tony Delk (left) and Walter McCarty (right) provided UK with the senior leadership it desperately needed.

cats before giving way to more experienced players.

Walter McCarty was a 6-10, 230-pound senior who moved into the starting lineup early in the season. Walter was very quick and fast for his size and could shoot from the perimeter with the best of them. He was also a very solid player on the inside.

Anthony Epps, a 6-2, 182-pound junior guard, was solid in every phase of the game. He could run the ball club with finesse. Pitino said of Epps, "He knows how to make other people better. He is a winner." Anthony was at his best when the game was on the line and he moved into the starting lineup early in the season as well.

Jared Prickett was expected to be available for his senior year and the 6-9, 235-pound forward was on hand after undergoing knee surgery the previous summer. Jared played in five games before the injury proved too much and he applied for a medical hardship. It was granted and he sat out the remainder of the season.

As the season progressed, the starting five shaped up with McCarty at center, Delk and Epps at the guards and Walker and Anderson at forwards. Even without Prickett, the Cats had great depth headed by Pope coming in as the sixth man. Pitino could also call on Jeff Sheppard, Allen Edwards, Turner, Mercer, Cameron Mills and Mohammed, even though Mills and Mohammed would see more action with the junior varsity. Pitino was blessed with a deep roster. "As deep as I've ever seen," he said. "Many times in our practices our second unit would beat our first unit."

After defeating Maryland in the Tip-Off Classic, the Cats traveled to the Great Eight in Auburn Hills, Michigan, to face Massachusetts. Coach John Calipari used only seven players but with the great Marcus Camby pouring in 32 points, UMass toppled the Cats, 92-82.

Pitino has always preached that a team can learn from its losses. "We learned two things," he said. "I was trying to play the most talented five people together. I realized we were not the best team playing the most talented athletes but we were better with Anthony Epps at the point and turning Tony loose to score at the two guard. Camby took advantage of the double-down by taking us on and scoring a lot. When you double-down, you're trying to get the man to pass and not shoot. When you trap-down, you're going all-out for a steal. We were trapping-down on the big men from that game on."

Pitino got them rolling again. The Cats ran off eight straight non-conference wins which included victories over Indiana, Louisville and the championship of the Holiday Classic in New York.

After easy SEC wins over South Carolina and Ole Miss, the Cats left for Starkville, Mississippi, for what was expected to be a showdown in the early conference race.

"We were driving to the game and our bus driver said he had never seen anything like it," Pitino said. "The cars were lined up

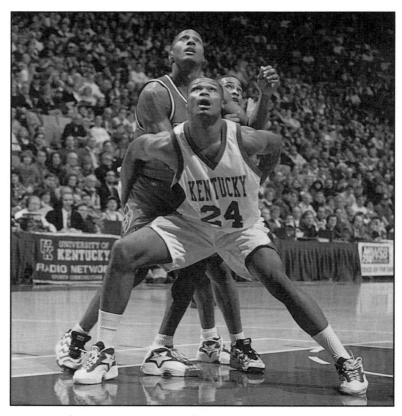

Just a sophomore, Antoine Walker played like a seasoned veteran and developed into the cornerstone of Kentucky's team.

for miles. The students were sleeping outside for the first time in MSU history. They expected to beat us."

Mississippi State had a fine team led by Erick Dampier and Dontaé Jones. The Bulldogs were ranked No. 12 and were picked to win the SEC's Western Division.

Walker led the Kentuckians with 16 points and Anderson came off the bench to score 12 as the Wildcats rolled to an unexpectedly easy victory, 74-56.

"We came out and dominated the game and took the crowd out of it," Pitino said. "The place was empty the final 10 minutes of play."

The Cats beat Tennessee, then went to Baton Rouge, Louisiana, for what Pitino thought would be a war with LSU. It was Kentucky's first trip to LSU since 1994, when UK orchestrated an amazing comeback from 31 points down with 15 minutes remaining in one of the most miraculous games ever played. The Cats finally prevailed, 99-95. Pitino thought LSU would use that game from two years before to motivate the team. Dale Brown would have them ready ... loaded for bear.

The day before the game, Rick went to the blackboard at practice and went over all the last-minute situations. He told the team what the Cats would do if they were up one or down by three and so on. He told the team this game would "go right down to the wire."

Kentucky came out smoking and totally overwhelmed the Bayou Tigers. By halftime, Kentucky had scored an incredible 86 points, a school and SEC record, to lead the Tigers at the intermission, 86-42. Just before the first half came to an end, Pitino's top aide, Jim O'Brien, turned to Rick and said, "Can you believe this? Thank God we went over those last-minute situations."

Pitino was stymied about what to say to his troops back in the dressing room. He stood before the group and said, "I told you guys this was going to be a close game." They all had a good laugh. The team didn't coast in the second half, and Kentucky won a lopsided decision, 129-97.

The meeting with Arkansas in Rupp Arena, February 11, 1996, was bathed in controversy. The Wildcats would defeat the Razorbacks for the first time in regular season play since Arkansas joined the SEC, 88-73. But the Cats broke out their new denim uniforms for that game, and all hell broke loose. Billy Packer, who was announcing the game on TV, said the uniforms looked like "Carolina Blue," and that didn't set well with UK fans. They just flat out didn't like the new look. "I've never seen so much controversy over uniforms in my life," Pitino said. "I just said you dress your children and we'll dress our own." As Kentucky kept winning, the mention of denim decreased dramatically.

On Senior Night, March 2, 1996, Kentucky defeated Vanderbilt to cap a remarkable 26-1 season but, even more amazing, the Cats became the first team in 40 years to go through the South-eastern Conference schedule undefeated. Pitino said, "I didn't think it was possible."

Rick had never lost an SEC Tournament game since coming to Kentucky and the Wildcats were favored to make it five championships in a row when the league teams gathered at the Superdome in New Orleans. Kentucky breezed past Florida and Arkansas to face Mississippi State in the final game.

Kentucky's shot selection left a lot to be desired and the fire had gone out of their defense. State walked off the court the winner, 84-73.

"I benched Antoine Walker because I saw some signs of the North Carolina game by other people," Rick told me. "I benched him and I said 'this is not going to happen again.'"

Pitino again embraced the loss. He thought it was the jolt his team needed to get back to doing the things that had been winning for them. "I knew we would get the eye of the tiger back again."

The Wildcats used a big second-half blitz to roll over San Jose State in the NCAA Tournament's first round of the Midwest Regional in Dallas.

In the second round, Kentucky again turned up the heat in the second half to beat Virginia Tech and advance to the Sweet 16 in Minneapolis. The final score was 84-60.

Kentucky advanced to the Elite Eight of the NCAA Tournament by eliminating Utah, 101-70.

The knock on Kentucky since Camby had his way with the Wildcats in the UMass game was that the Cats couldn't handle a multi-dimensional big man. Against Wake Forest in the Midwest Regional finals, Kentucky would face one of the premier centers in the college game in Tim Duncan. Pitino had learned from the earlier loss to UMass that the Wildcats would have to trap-down on a talented post player like Duncan, and Walker and McCarty did the

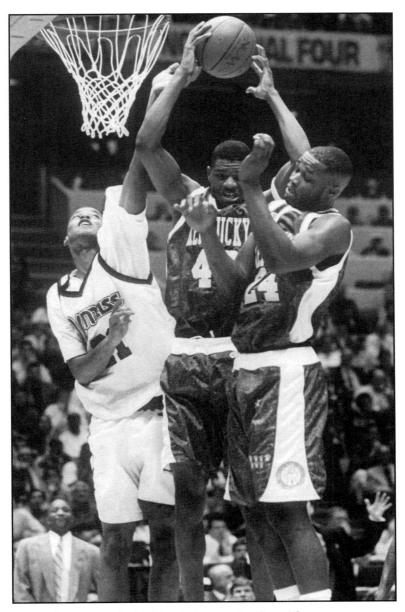

Kentucky surrounded UMass' Marcus Camby with two men throughout its NCAA semifinal game with the Minutemen, and it paid off with a seven-point victory.

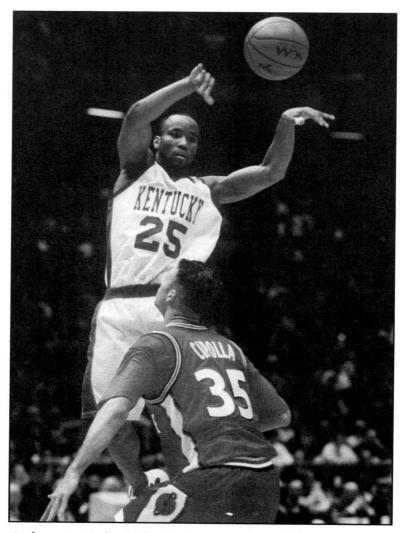

Anthony Epps' play in the Final Four was superb. The junior guard amassed 11 assists and a mere two turnovers.

lion's share of the trapping. They were so effective that Duncan attempted only three field goals in the first half, going 0 of 3. Kentucky's offense was in high gear and the Cats had a commanding 38-19 lead at the half. They were on their way to an 83-63 blowout of a fine Wake Forest team and its All-American center. Kentucky was so dominating in the Midwest Regional that four Wildcats — Delk, Anderson, Epps and Walker — were all named to the All-Regional team.

"That was as well-played basketball game as I've ever seen," Pitino said. "Not only did we attack offensively, but that's about as well as any team can play defensively." The Cats were headed for New Jersey and the Final Four.

At the Meadowlands, Kentucky was to meet one of the two teams that had beaten the Wildcats in the semifinals. UMass, with its Player of the Year, Marcus Camby, stood between the Cats and the championship game.

"I thought there were two great basketball teams in the country that year," Pitino said. "UMass and ourselves. I thought we had a devastating defense and an explosive offense. UMass was one of the best half-court teams both offensively and defensively. I felt good about our chances because I didn't think UMass could beat Kentucky twice because we had too much talent."

The pollsters agreed with Pitino that UMass and Kentucky were the best two teams in college basketball. As they lined up for the semifinal in the sports complex at the Meadowlands, UMass was ranked No. 1, Kentucky No. 2 in the nation. The two teams got ready to meet for the second time that season.

"The obvious thing was that we had to do a better job of shutting down Marcus Camby," Pitino said. He also felt that Tony Delk could be a key weapon coming off screens for his outside shots or taking the man guarding him down close to the basket to post up on him. "Delk was a great low-post player," Rick pointed out, "because he had this tremendous wingspan for a player his size."

A great game was expected between the No. 1 and No. 2 ranked teams, and the Minutemen and the Wildcats didn't disappoint. Delk wasn't getting open for the three-point shot, which stymied part of the UK attack, but the other strategy to get him on the low post worked like a charm. His 12 first-half points led the Cats to an

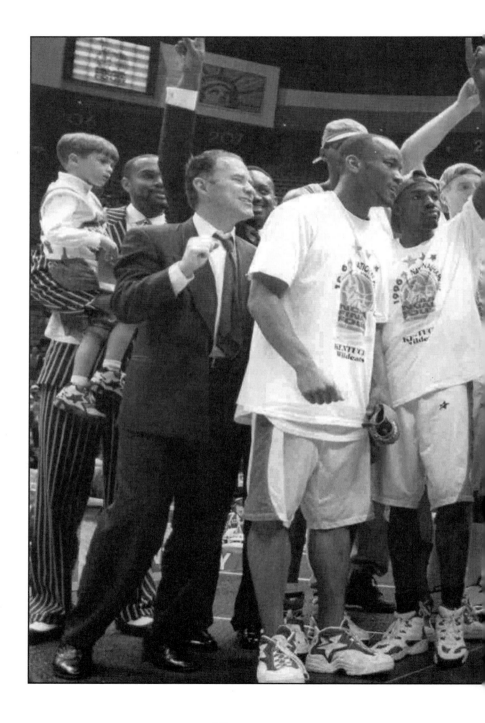

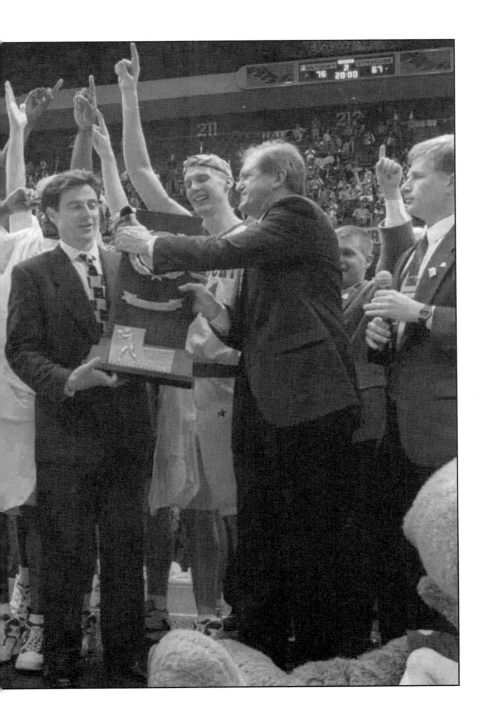

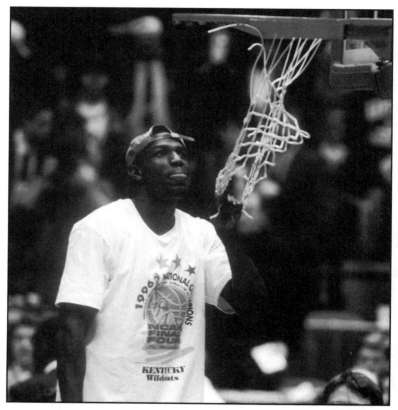

Final Four Most Outstanding Player Tony Delk culminated his UK career with a national title.

eight-point lead at the intermission, 36-28. Early in the second half, Kentucky pushed its lead to 15, 43-28. UMass wasn't about to roll over and play dead. The Minutemen stormed back and when the scoreboard showed 4:04 to play, Kentucky led by only three, 63-60. Camby fouled Mark Pope and the big senior was perfect for two at the charity line. Walker added another point from the free-throw line and Sheppard broke loose following a UMass turnover for a big dunk as the Cats pulled back out to an eight-point lead, 68-60. The clock showed 3:04 left to play.

The Minutemen mounted their last big charge and with 1:42 remaining had cut Kentucky's lead to four, 71-67. Anderson scored two free throws for the Wildcats and Edgar Padilla nailed a three-pointer for UMass to once again cut the Kentucky lead to three, 73-70. Pope, who was a perfect 6 of 6 from the charity line, hit his last two free throws and Walker got loose for a jam to seal the Kentucky victory. The Cats moved to the final game with an 81-74 win. Despite missing five minutes in the second half with leg cramps, Tony Delk led the Cats with 20 points. Two great basketball teams had played their guts out and both were exhausted at the end.

Pitino hoped that Mississippi State would defeat Syracuse in the other semifinal. Not just because State was from the Southeastern Conference, but Rick thought Kentucky would have a better shot at defeating the Bulldogs.

"Syracuse was the worst possible match-up for us," he said. "They were going to play zone and that was going to take the emotion and intensity out of the game. We were more tired, mentally and physically, than we had been all season and sometimes, against a man-to-man, a tired team can get the adrenaline flowing. But against a zone, it's slower paced and harder to get going."

Early in Pitino's career he had been an assistant to Jim Boeheim at Syracuse. The two coaches who would meet for the championship were friends and each was looking for his first title.

Kentucky had been so fatigued on the Sunday after the UMass game that Pitino was concerned.

"We had expended so much energy in the UMass game and we were very tired," he said. "We had been on an emotional high like you've never seen." On Monday night, he called the players together just before they left the dressing room and told them, "You were tired yesterday, but now you must muster up all your energy and focus in on every little detail in this basketball game in order to get a victory." He added, "I told them we had to have great shot selection against the Syracuse zone."

It was a nip-and-tuck war through most of the first half before Kentucky went on a 14-5 run to close the half and take a 42-33

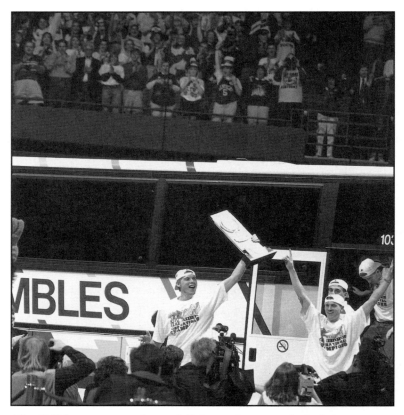

The Wildcats returned to a full Rupp Arena and Mark Pope showed the fans what they wanted.

lead. But nothing comes easy at the Final Four and behind the great play of Syracuse's John Wallace, the Orangemen cut Kentucky's lead to two points, 64-62, with 4:46 remaining. Delk was on target all evening, but this time he missed from three-point range. McCarty was there for the tip in. The next trip downcourt, Anderson nailed a three and Kentucky was ahead, 69-62. Syracuse was unable to meet the challenge and the Cats went on to post a 76-67 victory and win the NCAA Championship for the first time in 18 years.

"I had told our players to take only good shots. And they did. But we had won the championship shooting only 38 percent, which goes to show you a championship team wins with its defense. We missed 13 shots from within four feet."

Delk, who was named the Most Outstanding Player of the Final Four, tied the record for a championship game with seven three-pointers. He led the Cats with 24 points. Tony was a big part of the record 12 three-pointers the team scored in the championship game. "Tony Delk came up like the All-American he is," Pitino said.

Mercer came off the bench with fresh legs and had his best game of the season. The freshman forward scored 20 points, hitting 8 of 12 from the field, which included 3 of 4 from behind the three-point line. Boeheim said after the game, "Mercer was the guy who came in and hurt us."

Pitino said it felt wonderful to win the championship for the people of Kentucky and for the players. President Bill Clinton called shortly after the game to congratulate Pitino and the team. In May, the Cats would travel to the White House for a meeting with the President.

It had been a remarkable 10 months. There was an audience with the Pope in August 1995, the NCAA Championship the following April and a meeting with the President in May.

"From a spiritual sense, for a Catholic, nothing can be more fulfilling than meeting the Pope," Pitino said. "From a professional standpoint, nothing can be more fulfilling than winning the NCAA Championship and going to the White House to celebrate the championship season."

Rick says he'll never forget the reception back in jam-packed Rupp Arena following the NCAA Tournament. As they raised the banner reading, "NCAA CHAMPIONS, 1996," and Rick saw his players and family standing there and they were playing the song, "We are the Champions," he thought back over his seven years as the UK coach — from "Pitino's Bombinos" to the NCAA Champions. He thought to himself, "All this hard work was for one reason and that was for an entire state to be proud of its basketball team."

Rick Pitino almost lost it.

The Golden Year

Adolph Rupp put his greatest team together for the 1947-48 season, but it took a major world war, some changes in the college rules and nine long years to fashion a team that would be known as the "Fabulous Five."

The starters were Cliff Barker, Kenny Rollins, Alex Groza, Ralph Beard and Wallace "Wah Wah" Jones.

Barker was the first to arrive in Wildcat country. His high school coach, Kenneth Sigler, brought Cliff to Lexington from Yorktown, Indiana, for a tryout, which was legal and widely practiced in those days. Rupp was not impressed and Barker returned home disappointed. Coach Sigler apparently was quite a talker because he kept pleading Barker's case and Coach Rupp relented, offering Barker a scholarship. Barker enrolled in the fall of 1939, spent a year at Kentucky, then left for the Air Corps.

It was another two years before Kenny Rollins enrolled at UK. Rollins came out of Wickliffe High School in 1941. He was turned down for a scholarship after a tryout at Western Kentucky by Coach Ed Diddle. At the urging of friends in the western part of the state, Rupp invited Rollins to his tryout camp and, from a group of three dozen candidates, Rollins was one of five players at the camp who Rupp put on scholarship. He played with the freshman team

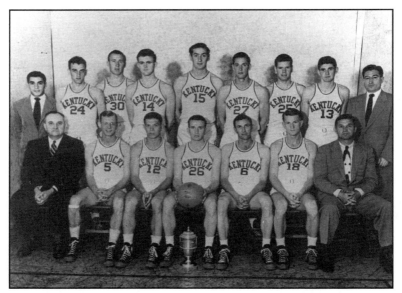

The 1947-48 Kentucky Wildcats. Front Row (L-R): Head Coach Adolph Rupp, Johnny Stough, Ralph Beard, Kenny Rollins, Cliff Barker, Dale Barnstable, Asst. Coach Harry Lancaster. Back Row: Mgr. Humzey Yessin, Garland Townes, Jim Jordan, Joe Holland, Alex Groza, Wallace Jones, Jim Line, Roger Day, Trainer Wilbert "Bud" Berger.

his first season then moved up to the varsity as a starter the next year. At the end of the 1942-43 season, Rollins was inducted into the Navy.

With America's entry into World War II after the Japanese bombed Pearl Harbor December 7, 1941, some players had a brief career before being drafted for military service. The manpower shortage became so critical that the national rules were changed to allow freshmen to play with the varsity. For the 1943-44 season, freshman Bob Brannum led the team in scoring and made the All-American team. He led the Cats to a third-place finish in the National Invitation Tournament before being drafted into the Army.

The third member of the "Fabulous Five" arrived in 1944 in the person of 6-4 1/2 Alex Groza from Martins Ferry, Ohio. Alex had hoped to follow his older brother, Walt, to Ohio State but the Buckeyes showed no interest. Kentucky was the only school that offered

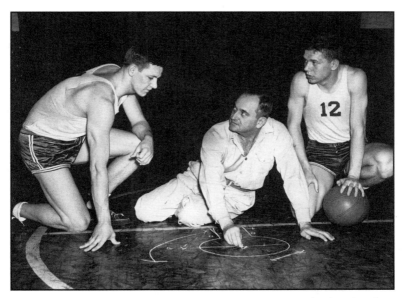

Two of the Commonwealth of Kentucky's greatest high school players of all-time, Wallace "Wah Wah" Jones (left) and Ralph Beard, receive instruction from Adolph Rupp.

a scholarship, and he played in only 11 games his first year before the Army called. He led the team in scoring and the Wildcats were undefeated when Groza departed.

The final two members of the "Fabulous Five" came aboard in 1945 when Rupp signed two of the greatest high school stars Kentucky has ever produced, Ralph Beard and Wallace "Wah Wah" Jones.

Jones became "Wah Wah" early in life when a younger sister, Jackie, couldn't quite pronounce Wallace. He was a legend while at Harlan High School, being named All-State in football his final two years and pitching the Green Dragons to the state baseball tournament twice. But it was the sport of basketball where he established a national reputation by scoring a record 2,398 points during his four years at Harlan. In 1944, Wah's junior year, he led the Dragons to the state championship.

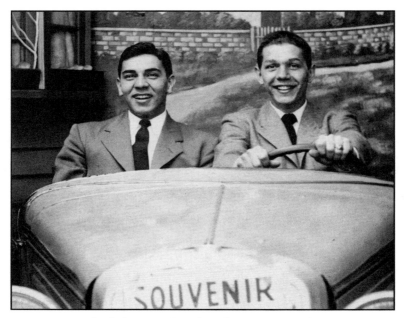

*Humzey Yessin (left), UK's head student manager, became a
fixture of UK basketball during the Golden Era, and Ralph Beard.*

Jones almost became a Tennessee Volunteer. Wah and Humzey
Yessin, a guard on the Harlan team, had almost agreed to join the
Vols but told some influential Tennessee boosters that they had to
return home to get their clothes. They were given the keys to a car
and headed for Harlan when Jones suggested they stop by Middles-
boro to visit Edna Ball (the future Mrs. Wallace Jones), who was a
student at UK. Edna, along with the help of her father and brother,
persuaded Jones to change his mind and matriculate to Kentucky.
Yessin got the dubious honor of taking the car back to Knoxville and
decided to join his old teammate at UK. Humzey would become
the team manager at Kentucky for the next four years.

Beard was an outstanding athlete at Male High School in
Louisville. He was an All-State halfback on the football team and
an outstanding open-field runner. He was a star second baseman
and the state champion half-miler on the track team. Beard led his

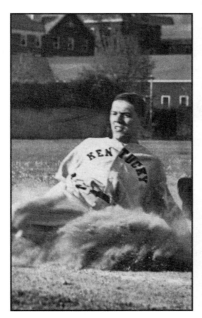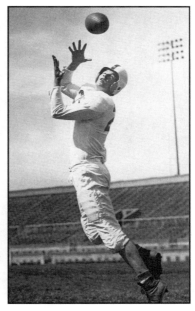

***Ralph Beard (left) and Wallace Jones were both multi-sport
athletes while at UK.***

basketball team in scoring for four straight years and was named to
the All-State team two years. During his senior season, Ralph led
Male to the state high school championship.

Oddly enough, both Beard and Jones went to Kentucky on football scholarships and made the starting 11 their freshmen year.
Jones went on to make All-Conference that season, but Beard's career was cut short when he separated both shoulders during the
fourth game of the season. Despondent, Beard decided to quit
school and return home to Louisville where some friends of the
University of Louisville talked him into transferring. Since Beard in-
tended to play basketball too, he went back to UK to tell Rupp of
his decision. Ralph told me recently that Rupp looked straight at
him and said, "Son, I don't know why you would want to go to that
damned normal school (teachers' college), but I can assure you we
still plan to play our schedule." Ralph's high school coach, Paul

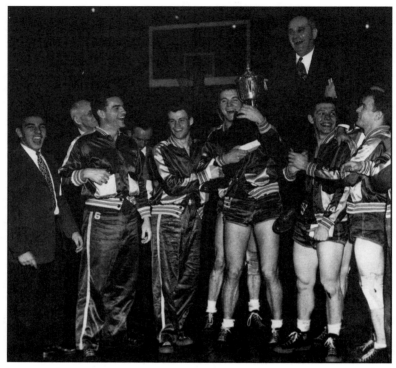

The Wildcats gave their coach a ride after winning the
1946 National Invitation Tournament title.

Jenkins, told him he would be making a terrible mistake and Ralph returned to the Wildcats.

With Beard and Jones both starting as freshmen, the Wildcats had a marvelous year. Jack Parkinson was the leading scorer on the season as the Cats lost only twice — at Temple and to Notre Dame in Louisville. Kentucky breezed through the SEC Tournament and then got revenge against Temple in a postseason game in Louisville. The Cats accepted a bid to the NIT.

"The NIT was a lot bigger back then than the NCAA," said Beard. "Coach Rupp told us the NCAA had a bunch of 'YMCA teams.'" Rupp might have exaggerated that to some extent because both tournaments drew some strong teams in 1946.

Kentucky defeated Arizona handily in the first game but had to score the last eight points against West Virginia to beat the Mountaineers, 59-51. The Cats had a war with Rhode Island in the finals and with the game on the line, Beard stepped to the free throw line and hit the winning basket as Kentucky prevailed, 46-45. Kentucky and Rupp had won their first national title. The players hoisted Rupp to their shoulders and carried him in triumph to the dressing room.

Rupp had watched as his players departed for military service, but for the 1946-47 season, his players came marching back home.

Rupp had nine lettermen back from that 28-2 team that had won the NIT. The players returning from military service were even more impressive. Brannum and Groza, who were teammates on the Fort Hood, Texas, team, rejoined the Cats. Brannum was an All-American two years earlier at Kentucky and Groza, who had spurted to 6-7 while in the service, had been named the best player in the armed services. Barker was back after spending almost two years in a Prisoner of War camp. Dale Barnstable had his Navy discharge and returned. Jim Jordan joined the team after twice being named to the All-American team at North Carolina Pre-Flight [School].

At the beginning of practice for the 1946-47 season, Rupp had more than 40 players trying to make the squad, including a pair of very talented freshmen, Dale Barnstable and Jim Line. No matter what the players' status had been before, each had to compete all over again for a place on the squad.

Rupp tinkered with his starting lineup much of the season but with Groza, Beard, Rollins, Jones and Joe Holland leading the scoring, the Cats posted a brilliant 34-3 worksheet. They were upset by Oklahoma A&M (now Oklahoma State) in the Sugar Bowl Tournament and dropped a decision to DePaul in Chicago. That team was so deep that Rupp had to make some difficult choices when the Southeastern Conference permitted him to dress only 10 players for the league tournament in Louisville.

Yessin, the popular team manager all during the golden era, said

51

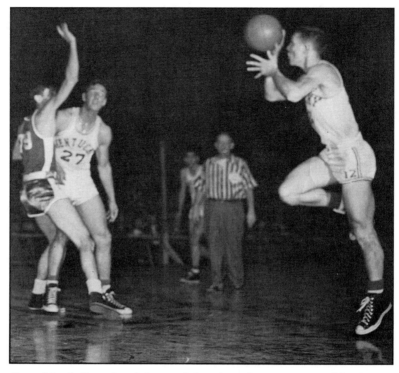

Beard took Rupp's advice and developed a potent outside shot.

to understand the depth of that team, "Three All-Americans didn't even make the traveling squad. Brannum, Parkinson and Jordan didn't even get to suit up. They went to the tournament and watched from the stands."

Kentucky had a cake-walk through the SEC Tournament and defeated Temple in a postseason game in Louisville and headed for New York to defend its NIT title.

The Cats squeezed out a 63-62 win over Long Island, then took a comfortable decision versus North Carolina State. In the finals, the Cats were stunned by Utah, 49-45, as Utah's Wat Misaka held Beard without a field goal.

Despite being named the outstanding player to see action in Madison Square Garden that year, Beard was devastated with his performance. He went to Rupp to ask what he could do to improve his game and the Kentucky coach told Ralph that he needed to develop an outside shot.

Yessin was Beard's college roommate and he said, "Ralph had such speed and quickness, he depended on that to drive to the basket for his shots. It had been enough to make him an All-American. Misaka was a Japanese-American and he played a smart game against (the taller) Beard. He played off Ralph and cut off his drives."

Nobody wanted to be a better basketball player than Ralph Beard and he took his coach's advice to heart. Yessin told me recently, "Ralph and I were teammates on the Kentucky baseball team and that spring, almost every day, we went to Alumni Gym and he shot hundreds of two-handed set shots. The next season he was one of the best outside shooters in the country."

The Fabulous Five

Harry Lancaster's partiality might have been showing when he said, "The 1947-48 Kentucky Wildcats team, in my opinion, was the best college basketball team that has ever set foot in a gymnasium." But Lancaster was the assistant coach at Kentucky while the Wildcats won four of their six championships. We do have to give some credence to his opinion. It was an opinion he shared with his old boss. Rupp believed that the "Fabulous Five" was his best in the 41 seasons he put a Kentucky team on the court.

Kentucky ran off with a seven-game winning streak without the services of Jones, as Rupp experimented with his starting lineup. Each season, because of football, Jones had to retake his starting job. Each season he was able to do so.

He was still coming off the bench when the Wildcats traveled to Philadelphia to face Temple. Jones was nursing an ankle injury and didn't get into the game as Temple handed the Cats their first defeat, 60-59.

"I always thought that Coach Rupp resented my playing foot-

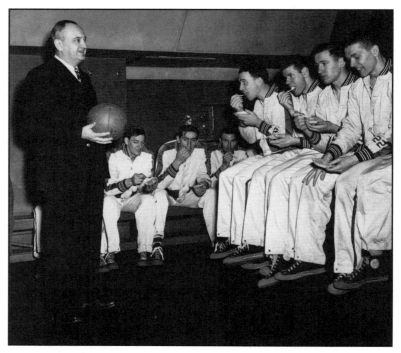

Coach Rupp looks on as his Wildcats indulge in some ice cream.

ball," Jones told me. "I was the only one playing both sports and I was a little behind the others when I reported for basketball, but the week before that Temple game I had practiced full-speed."

After that one-point loss to the Owls, Yessin went to Rupp's hotel room to pick up the players' meal money for the next day.

"Coach Rupp was lying there in bed with those bright red pajamas talking with several members of the press. They were all wondering why we had lost. He asked me, 'Humzey, why do you think we lost?' I told him I thought we should have played Jones."

Yessin said that Rupp sat straight up in bed and told him to go get George Hukle and bring him back to his room. Hukle was the equipment manager but he also kept all the statistics for the Wildcats. Yessin said he awakened Hukle and the two went to Rupp's room. The Kentucky coach took the stats and began to compare

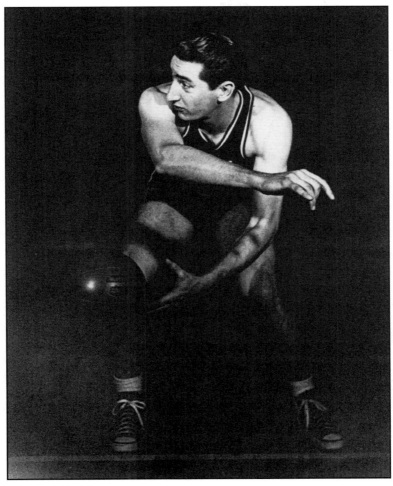

***During the Golden Era, Alex Groza was one of the nation's best
post players.***

what Jones had done in the games to that of his opponent. Jones
didn't fare too well in the comparison.

"He just folded those sheets," Yessin said, "and with a little smile
on his face he said, 'You damn Harlan people just stick together!'"
Case closed.

Whether Yessin's suggestion to Rupp had any bearing on it we'll

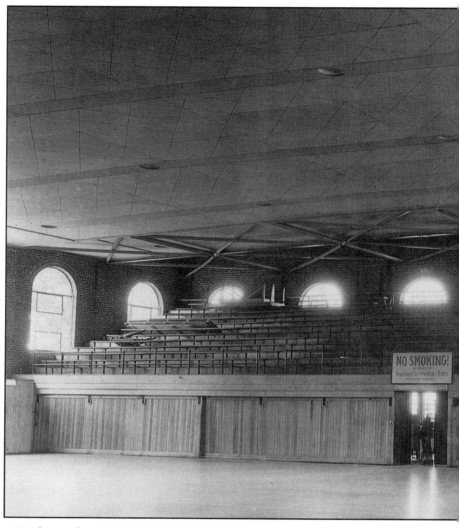

UK's home from 1924-50 was Alumni Gym. The building could hold 2,800 patrons and was one of the greatest settings for basketball of its time.

never know, but Jones received considerable playing time in the next game. Wah scored 16 points as the Wildcats defeated St. John's in Madison Square Garden.

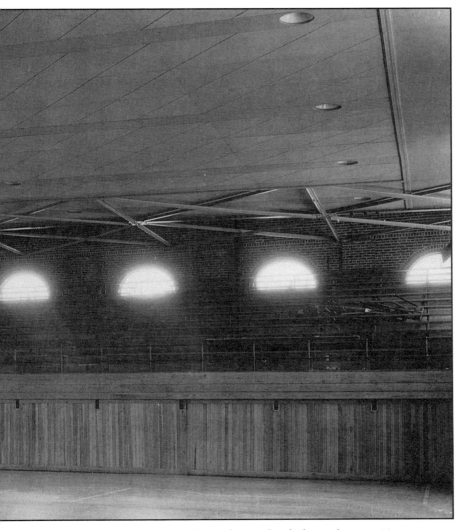

Rupp had most of the players back from the previous season. Brannum, who was getting little playing time, was an exception as he decided to transfer to Michigan State.

"He damn near beat us too," Beard told me. On January 10, Kentucky prevailed in a hard-fought battle on the road over Michigan State, 47-45.

Rupp changed his starting lineup throughout the season and it wasn't until January 12, 1948, that the Kentucky coach stood in the dressing room and announced that Groza, Beard, Rollins, Barker and Jones would be his starters against Ohio University. He couldn't have known it at the time, but he had put together one of the greatest college teams of all time. Groza, Beard, Jones and Barker were juniors. Rollins was a senior.

Had it not been for World War II, Barker and Rollins would have graduated from UK before Jones and Beard graduated from high school.

Barker was the old man of the group, turning 27 during the season. He had been shot down with his B-17 bomber crew over Germany and while he was a Prisoner of War, Barker got a volleyball out of a Red Cross package and became extremely adept with his ball handling. When he rejoined the Wildcats, he didn't score a lot of points, but he was a magician with the basketball. Jones said Barker was the first player he ever saw who could look one way and throw a perfect pass in the opposite direction. He was a pioneer of the "look-away pass."

"You had to stay alert when Barker had the ball," Jones said. "He'd fire you a pass and hit you in the head with it." He was also a fine defensive player and was always assigned to the other team's best scoring forward.

As good as Barker was defensively, the best defensive player on the team was Kenny Rollins. He was the team captain and provided great leadership. Today, he would be called a point guard, as he started every play in the half-court offense. Lancaster said of Rollins, "He had the best mind of any player we ever had." Yessin also had high praise for Kenny, calling him, "the best defensive player I ever saw."

Groza was just a phenomenal basketball player. At 6-7, he was a tall player for his time but by no means was he among the biggest centers in the college game. He had already been named to the All-American team and could play both ends of the court. Groza had a terrific shooting touch and was a tremendous rebounder. He usu-

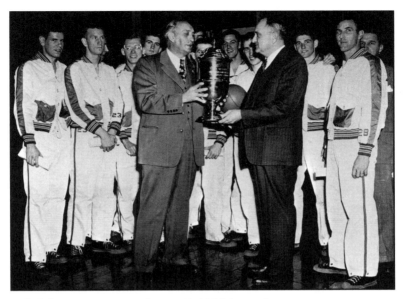

Adolph Rupp accepts the 1948 NCAA trophy.

ally triggered the fast break and could run the court with uncanny speed. He had great self-confidence and was close to unstoppable in the pivot.

Beard had blinding speed and was a superbly conditioned athlete. "He could play the whole game at top speed," Jones told me, "and not even be breathing deeply at the end." A tougher competitor never lived than the 5-10 guard. Beard, like Groza, had already been named an All-American. Lancaster said of him, "Inch for inch and pound for pound, Ralph Beard was the greatest basketball player I ever saw." Beard told me that in those days, basketball was the most important thing in his life.

Jones was perhaps the best pure athlete on the team. He was the last UK player, in my mind, to excel at both football and basketball. He made All-SEC and All-American in each sport. At 6-5, 200-pounds, Jones was a rough, tough competitor. He had a good two-hand overhead shot from the side and was rugged under the boards. The tougher the going, the tougher Jones played. He could play either forward or center but it was at the forward position that he made his best contribution to the "Fabulous Five."

The "Fabulous Five" was not an overnight success. Rupp had been building the Wildcat program from the day he arrived in Lexington in 1930. Kentucky had winning programs before he came, but Rupp installed a fast-break style of basketball that was new to the South. After Kentucky became dominant in its region, Rupp took the team outside the area, playing Notre Dame, some of the top teams in the Big Ten and once a year he would invade the East to face strong teams in that locality.

Rupp drove himself and his players hard. He was very demanding and his practices were short but very intense. If a player made a mistake, that player was corrected on the spot. Winning was everything to him. If I wanted to get him riled up during an interview, all I had to do was ask him about Grantland Rice's famous poem that read, "It mattered not if you won or lost but how you played the game." With a trace of anger in his voice, Rupp would respond, "Well, if it doesn't matter whether you win or lose, why do they keep score? It makes all the difference in the world." Rupp was so successful that he drew some criticism from among some of his coaching colleagues. Some were no doubt jealous of his domination of the game in the SEC. He seemed to be impervious to criticism but he demanded, and usually received, winning performances from his teams. "I am not engaged in a popularity contest," he said. "I want to win."

No one seems exactly sure how the nickname the "Fabulous Five" came about. Both Beard and Jones think it was given to the team by Larry Boeck, a sportswriter for *The Courier-Journal*. In reality, to call that 1947-48 Kentucky team the "Fabulous Five" was a misnomer. Rupp had a deep bench. Holland, a sometime starter, was a returning All-Conference player. Even though Brannum had transferred, Parkinson and Jordan gave Rupp two All-Americans on the bench. Barnstable, Line and Johnny Stough were quality players who Rupp could summon from his bench as well.

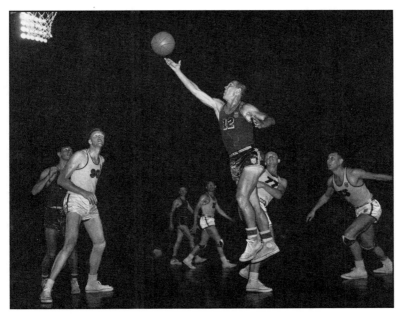

Ralph Beard drives the lane against the Phillips Oilers during the final Olympic exhibition game, played outdoors at Stoll Field.

Following the loss to Temple, the Cats stumbled only once more during the season, losing at Notre Dame. Kentucky took its No. 1 national ranking and headed to New York for its first NCAA Tournament engagement.

First up for the Cats in Madison Square Garden was Columbia. Rupp was one of the pioneers in scouting an opponent and despite Columbia's gaudy 21-1 record, his scouts figured the Cats should easily handle the Lions. That proved accurate as Kentucky breezed to a 76-53 win.

The scouting report on Holy Cross, UK's next opponent, was quite different. The scouts predicted that it would take a great game by the Cats to win. It certainly didn't figure to be a walk in the park and it wasn't. The Crusaders had won the NCAA title the previous year and rode an 18-game winning streak into the Garden. Holy Cross was led by George Kaftan and the great Bob Cousy. A hand-

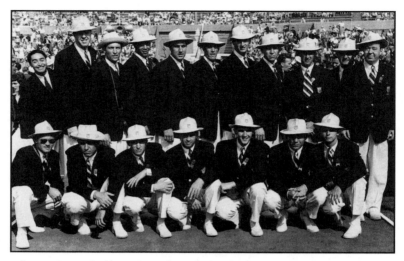

The 1948 United States Olympic basketball team in London during the games' opening ceremonies.

painted bed sheet fluttered from the rafters proclaiming Cousy "the greatest player in the world." Rupp believed stopping Cousy was the key to winning the game and charged Rollins with that difficult assignment. Kenny was up to the job. When Rollins left late in the game, Cousy had three points, all on free throws. Groza was too much for Kaftan, scoring 23 points and controlling the boards. Kentucky beat Holy Cross, 60-52, to win the Eastern Regional. "After the game," Jones told me, "somebody brought that bed sheet and gave it to Rollins."

The final game against West Regional champion Baylor saw Kentucky win in a breeze, 58-42, to claim its first NCAA Championship.

"The statistics from that team are misleading," Yessin told me. "If you came to our games during the halftime intermission, a lot of times you wouldn't even see the starters."

Lancaster said the "Fabulous Five" was so superior to the teams they played, "I can recall several times during the halftime, Adolph would order the starters to get dressed and not even show up for the second half."

Four days after winning the NCAA Tournament, Kentucky took part in the Olympic Trials to select a team to represent this country. To win the collegiate bracket Kentucky had to defeat Louisville and again take the measure of Baylor. Both wins came easily.

Then, the Cats had to face the powerful Phillips Oilers. Pro basketball was not what it is today and some of the top college stars had gravitated to the Oilers and the other AAU teams that offered work along with playing ball. The Oilers were headed by a seven-footer, Bob Kurland. In a game that the New York writers would call one of the best ever played in the Garden, the Oilers won 53-49. Under the guidelines used to select an Olympic team, the five starters from each team would make up the majority of players who would represent the USA. Oiler coach Bud Browning was named the head coach while Rupp was placed in the unaccustomed role of associate coach.

Rupp, publicly, was high in his praise of the Oilers calling them "the best team we faced all season." Ralph Beard remembers that right after the loss to the Oilers back in the UK dressing room, Rupp was less gracious, saying, "I want to thank you bastards for making me an assistant coach for the first time in my life."

Surprisingly, perhaps, Rupp and Browning got along well and their association became very close.

The team sailed to London on the U.S.S. America and the journey was enjoyed by the players.

"All of our Olympic athletes were on the ship," Jones said, "and we got to know a lot of them who competed in other sports. It was the first time most of us had ever been on a ship or traveled outside the country."

Because of the war, the Olympic Games were being held for the first time in a dozen years. The U.S. team won all eight of its games, most of them by lopsided scores. Jones and Beard agreed it was the biggest honor of their playing careers. To his dying day, Rupp said it was the highlight of his long coaching career.

"To watch our boys stand on that podium in London, England,

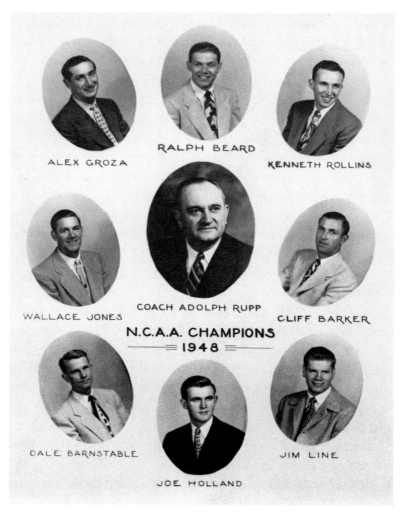

RALPH BEARD

ALEX GROZA

KENNETH ROLLINS

COACH ADOLPH RUPP

WALLACE JONES

CLIFF BARKER

N.C.A.A. CHAMPIONS
═ 1948 ═

DALE BARNSTABLE

JIM LINE

JOE HOLLAND

and watch them drape those gold medals around their necks while they played the national anthem, was my biggest thrill in sports."

The "Fabulous Five" was the first Kentucky basketball team I ever saw in person. I was a student at Centre College in Danville during those years and I was fortunate to have friends at UK who could come up with a ticket from time to time. They played their games in Alumni Gym, a 2,800-seat arena, and by the time the 1947-48 team came along, only a portion of the students were able

to attend the games. The general public had to be content to follow the Wildcats by radio or in the newspaper. That team was so
awesome that Big Blue fever really hit the Commonwealth. That
was the beginning of the mania that Kentuckians feel about their
team ... It exists to this very day.

The Second Time Around

If ever a man was born more superstitious, I never met him. Adolph Rupp relied heavily on trinkets that brought him good luck. Even if they didn't, he took no chances and acquired them for insurance.

Anytime I wanted to get his goat, all I had to do was begin telling him about a new superstition I had heard. He would throw up his hands, tell me to stop talking foolish and hurriedly walk away. Apparently, he felt he couldn't bear the burden of one more superstition.

He always carried a four-leaf clover and a buckeye in his pocket. On days the Cats played at home, he parked in the same place each time, took the same route to the gym, even stepped on the same manhole cover. For games on the road, after the pregame meal, he took a walk and looked for hair pins on the way. The more he found, the better his luck would be that night. Players had been known to salt a few along the way they knew he would be walking.

Rupp was known as the "Man in the brown suit." More than anything else, that came closest to being the colorful coach's trade-mark. It all started while Rupp was coaching at Freeport High School in Illinois. His team was doing well. He owned only one

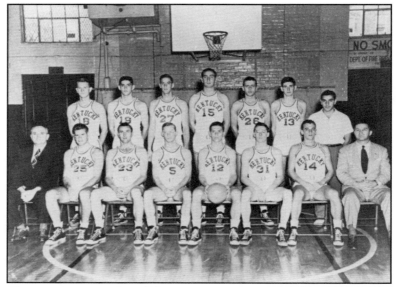

The 1948-49 Kentucky Wildcats. Front Row (L-R): Head Coach Adolph Rupp, Jim Line, Cliff Barker, John Stough, Ralph Beard, Joe B. Hall, Garland Townes, Asst. Coach Harry Lancaster. Back Row: Dale Barnstable, Walt Hirsch, Wallace Jones, Alex Groza, Bob Henne, Roger Day, Mgr. Humzey Yessin.

suit and it happened to be brown. Rupp decided it was time for a new suit and he bought a blue one.

"I made an auspicious entry into the gym that night and I thought I looked pretty spiffy in that blue suit," Coach Rupp told me. "I don't think anybody else noticed but that night we got the dickens beat out of us. I got to studying about that thing and decided that blue suit didn't help any. So, I went back to the old brown suit and we started winning again." Coach Rupp said he never wore anything but brown on the day of a game after that ill-fated experience with blue.

If Kentucky was winning during a tournament, Rupp liked to keep things as much the same as possible. After a win, he would go to his hotel room and wash out his socks so that he could wear that same pair again the next day. Why leave anything to chance?

With all of his superstitions in tow, Rupp faced the 1948-49 sea-

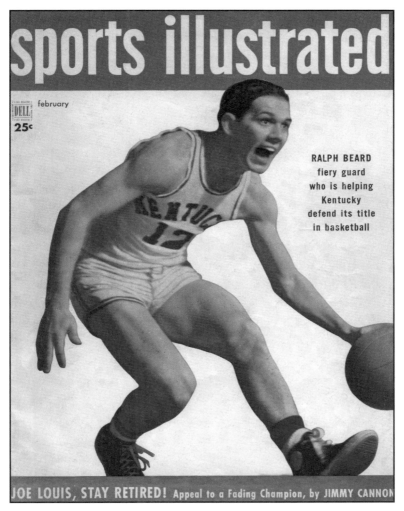

The February 1949 issue of Sports Illustrated depicted Ralph Beard as Kentucky prepared to defend its national title.

son with a lot of confidence. Why not? He had four starters back from the team that had won the NCAA Tournament the previous year and shared in the Olympic Gold Medal. Kenny Rollins had graduated and gone on to play professional basketball, but he was the only starter lost to the "Fabulous Five." Joe Holland and Jim Jor-

69

dan were the only other members of the squad who had played out their eligibility. Walt Hirsch and Joe B. Hall moved up to join the varsity. Hirsch would go on to contribute to UK's success. Hall, lacking playing time, would ask Rupp's help in transferring to Sewanee. He would make his contribution to the UK program in a different fashion several years later.

Rupp thought that his 1948-49 team could be even better than the "Fabulous Five" and they certainly looked the part at the start of the season. After exploding for four easy wins to begin the campaign, the Wildcats began their annual invasion of the East, first to Boston for a date with Holy Cross, then back to New York to meet St. John's.

The Boston Garden was packed with 14,000 fans as Kentucky faced Holy Cross. The two teams had met in the NCAA Tournament the previous season, with Kentucky coming away the winner. The Crusaders were primed for the Cats and it was a street-fight with Kentucky's Cliff Barker and Bob Cousy of Holy Cross actually getting into a fight.

Wah Jones fouled out late in the game and as he was sitting on the bench a fan was really heckling the Kentucky senior. As Jones turned the fan hit him in the face with a wadded-up cigarette package. Jones grabbed the man by the shirt with his left hand and delivered a hard right to the man's jaw. Harry Lancaster said "The man was lying on the floor and Wah was standing there holding the man's tie and shirt front in his left hand." Later, Lancaster himself became involved in some fisticuffs with a Holy Cross fan and made it two-for-two in Kentucky's favor. When order was finally restored, the Cats won a close 51-48 decision.

Two nights later, before a packed house in Madison Square Garden, the Cats made a shambles of St. John's, 57-30.

Kentucky sailed through the first eight games on the schedule before coming up short in the Sugar Bowl Tournament as St. Louis converted a tip-in on a missed free throw for a 42-40 decision. The Cats played poorly and Rupp was furious.

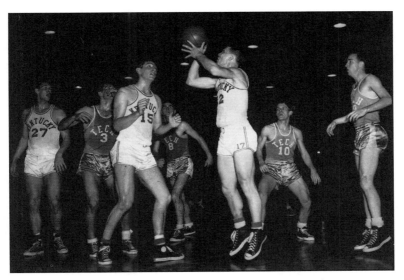

The "Fabulous Five" were no longer, but seniors Wah Jones (27), Alex Groza (15) and Ralph Beard (12) and the rest of the Wildcats continued to dominate the collegiate game.

The next time out, Kentucky edged an underdog, Bowling Green, in a game played at Cleveland, 63-61. To say that Rupp was disappointed in his team would be a gross understatement.

When he got his team back to Lexington, he put them through some of the most rugged practices any team ever had to endure. Rupp was not going to tolerate lackadaisical performances from his Wildcats. Lancaster said that for the remainder of that season the best games he watched were those played in Alumni Gym during the UK practices.

"When you could split the kind of talent we had into two teams," he said, "you really had a game in those scrimmages."

After the loss to St. Louis and the close call against Bowling Green, Kentucky righted its ship and sailed on through the regular season and the SEC Tournament without another loss.

Even though four starters were back from the "Fabulous Five," Kentucky adopted a different style of play during the 1948-49

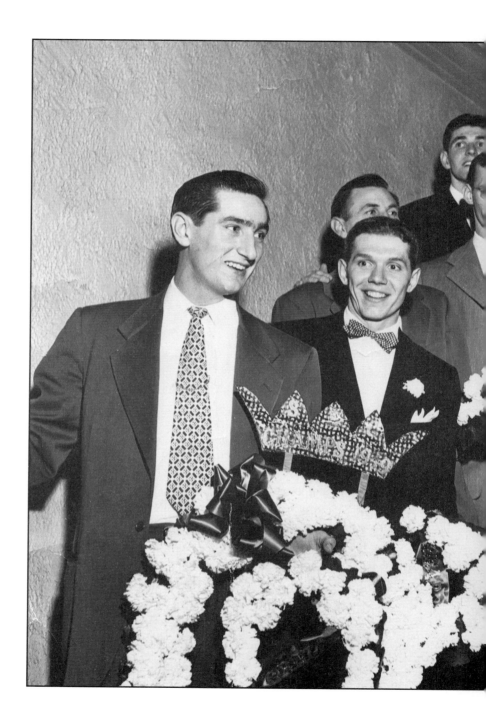

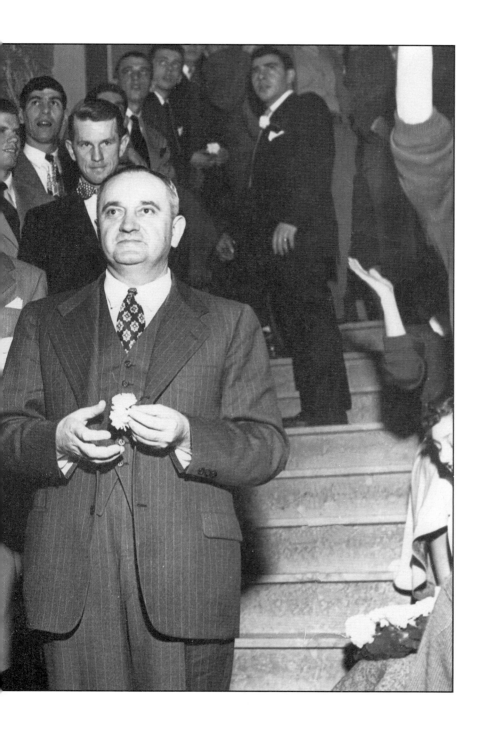

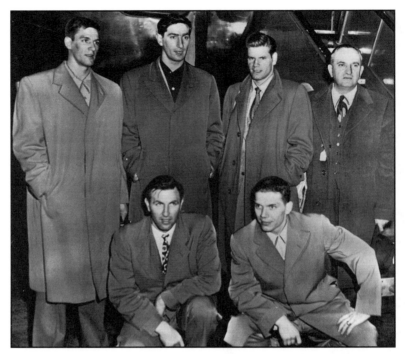

The Wildcats arrived in Seattle, Washington, to defend their
NCAA title. Front Row (l-r): Cliff Barker and Ralph Beard.
Back Row: Wah Jones, Alex Groza, Jim Line and Adolph Rupp.

season. From a balanced attack that featured Groza, Beard and Jones, the Cats were now focusing on Groza, without question the best center in college basketball. That season, Groza scored more points than Beard and Jones combined. The new plan had worked well and Kentucky was rewarded for a great season by being invited to take part in both the NIT and NCAA tournaments. It marked the first time a team would try to win both post-season classics in the same year.

Kentucky's first game in the NIT was a disaster. Loyola of Chicago upset the Cats, 67-56. Rupp had thought that Groza would have his way with Loyola's center, Jack Kerris. Groza, for some reason, didn't seem to have his heart in the game. He had four fouls on

Kerris at the half, but with the Kentucky bench screaming for Groza to take it to Kerris, it was Groza who fouled out.

Rupp and Lancaster agonized far into the night following that loss.

"Harry, what in the hell was wrong with Alex out there tonight?" he asked over and over. Lancaster had no answer to Rupp's questions. "It was two years later that we got our answer," Lancaster said. "Our players were shaving points."

It was a week later that Kentucky was scheduled for NCAA play back in Madison Square Garden. Rupp took his troops back to Lexington for some intense drills. "I spared no mercy," he said. As Coach Rupp was fond of saying, he took his players "to the woodshed." They took the train back to New York to face Villanova in the East Regional.

Kentucky played perhaps its best basketball of the season in the NCAA Tournament. With Groza scoring 30 points, the Cats easily dispatched of Villanova, 85-72. They came back in the second round and demolished a proud Illinois team, 76-47. Groza again led the rout with 27 points.

Between games in New York, Rupp sent Lancaster to Kansas City to scout the West Regional. Making frequent trips between the two cities, Lancaster watched Oklahoma A&M survive the closest game in the tournament by edging Wyoming, 40-39. Hank Iba then led his charges to the West Regional title by breezing past Oregon State, 55-30. Oklahoma A&M left for Seattle to await the Wildcats to battle for the NCAA Championship.

Lancaster flew back to New York to join the team and to give his scouting report on Oklahoma A&M to Rupp. Iba called Bob Harris "the best defensive center I ever coached," but Lancaster thought Harris would not be able to handle the more versatile Groza. "Get the ball to Groza," was Lancaster's basic scouting report.

On the train to Seattle, Rupp and Lancaster had plenty of time to hatch their battle plan. Rupp decided the best strategy would be to pass the ball to Jones' side of the floor and let Wah drive into the lane and dish the ball off to Groza.

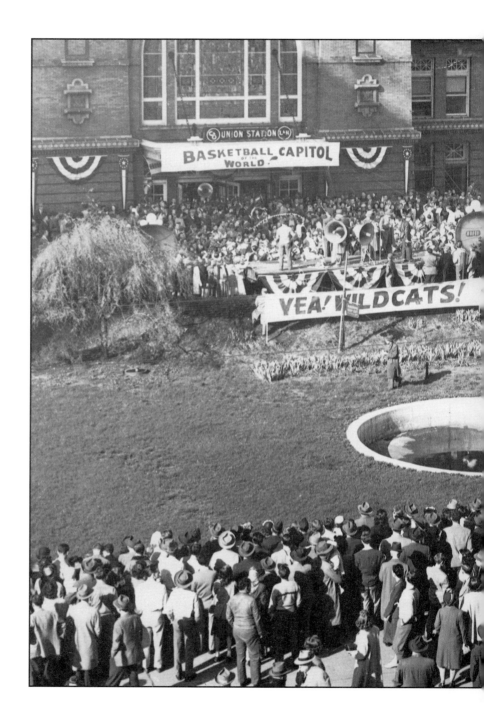

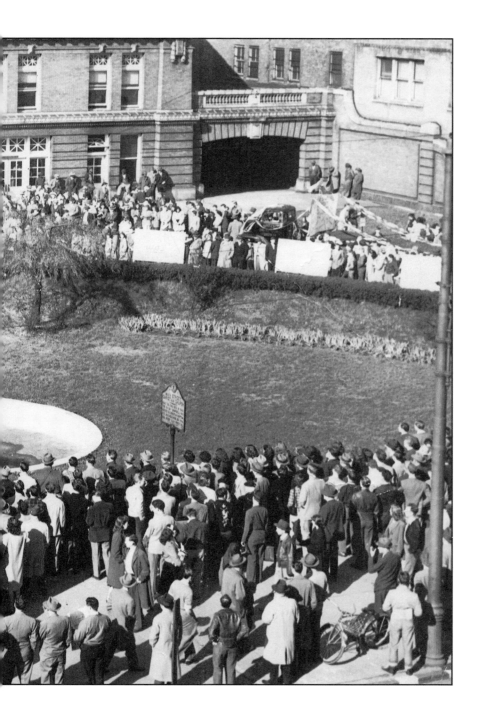

Kentucky was ranked No. 1 and Oklahoma A&M No. 2 as they prepared to meet at the University of Washington Pavilion. The two teams were a study in contrasts. Kentucky liked to fast-break, to run, run, run. A&M played a very deliberate, ball-control game. Both teams stressed defense. Rupp and Iba were both outstanding coaches who would rank among the best even today.

Kentucky arrived in Seattle with three All-Americans — Groza, Jones and Beard. In a team meeting, Coach Rupp mentioned all of his all-stars and according to Humzey Yessin, "Coach Rupp looked right at Barker and said, 'Cliff, I guess we'll just have to make you All-Fayette County.' " Everybody had a good laugh.

Kentucky proved to have the better game plan. Iba, who usually went with a sagging man-to-man defense, decided to play a straight man-to-man, feeling that Harris could handle Groza. It was a costly miscalculation.

Kentucky ran its game plan just the way Rupp had instructed the team. The ball went to Jones' side of the court and Wah drove by Jack Shelton. Jones said, "I was able to get the step on the man guarding me and Harris had to drop off Groza to pick me up. When I got the ball to Groza, Alex was wide open." Groza ripped A&M for 25 points as Kentucky won 46-36. For the second straight year, Groza was named the Most Outstanding Player in the NCAA Tournament but Lancaster said, "To my mind, Wah Jones was the most valuable player for us that night."

Kentucky became only the second team to win two NCAA titles. Ironically, the other was Oklahoma A&M, winners in 1945 and '46, with Iba on the bench.

Once Kentucky achieved a comfortable lead in the second half, the Cats abandoned their run-and-gun game to slow it down, much in A&M's style of play. Lancaster was to say, "You might say we beat the Aggies at their own game."

Kentucky had come to expect warm receptions back home after achieving a high accomplishment. For 1949, the Commonwealth had saved its best.

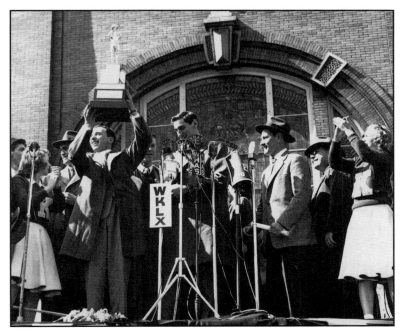

Alex Groza speaks to the crowd gathered to welcome home the 1949 NCAA Champions.

The biggest crowd to ever welcome the Wildcats showed up at Union Station in Lexington with life-size pictures of all the players and coaches.

Later, at "Wildcat Appreciation Day," they threw a big parade for the team before a crowd that was estimated at 25,000. Rupp announced that the jerseys of Beard, Barker, Groza and Jones would be retired, along with that of Rollins, who had graduated the year before. He had enshrined forever the "Fabulous Five."

I saw both the 1948 and '49 teams play at old Alumni Gym. The personnel was almost identical. Barker, Beard, Groza and Jones were starters on both teams. Dale Barnstable replaced Rollins on the 1949 team as a starter, until Rupp replaced Dale with Jim Line just before the NCAA Tournament. I know that Coach Rupp always considered the 1948 team the best he ever coached. Lancaster called it the "...best college basketball team that has ever set foot in a gymnasium." I confess that I, too, thought the '48 team was a tick better. In a conversation recently with Jones, Beard and Yessin, I asked their opinion and all three agreed.

"For some reason," Yessin told me, "that '48 team just had a better chemistry. Rollins was probably the key. With Kenny and Beard in the game, they could just destroy the guards on the other team."

Jones was of about the same opinion.

"I guess Rollins was the difference," he said. "We really missed his defense the next year."

Beard agreed that Rollins was the team's best defensive player, but he thought Kenny brought some other things to the table.

"He was our captain," Ralph said, "and Kenny was just a tremendous leader. He was what we called a first guard back then, which meant he started most of our plays. He was just a terrific all-around player."

With no more worlds to conquer in the collegiate field, the four seniors persuaded "Babe" Kimbrough, a former Lexington sports editor, to set up a barnstorming tour. The Kentucky players also persuaded Holland and Rollins to join their team. Calling themselves the Kentucky Olympians, the boys from Kentucky played 17 games all across Kentucky and parts of West Virginia, drawing overflow crowds everywhere.

Rollins was already playing pro basketball but Holland joined Barker, Beard, Groza and Jones to own their own franchise in the pro ranks. It was the first time players had owned a franchise and the first time all the players from one school had played on the same pro team. They called themselves the Indianapolis Olympians, and played their home games in the Hoosier capital city.

Beard and Jones were the only members of the "Fabulous Five" who had been together for four straight years at UK. Jones was justifiably proud of what they had accomplished.

"Beard and I," Jones said, "played on teams who won 130 games and lost only 10. We won an NIT and two NCAA championships. We won an Olympic gold medal and in four years, we never lost a home game or lost to a Southeastern Conference team anywhere in regular season or tournament play."

The "Fabulous Five" had a remarkable career, perhaps the brightest era in Kentucky Basketball.

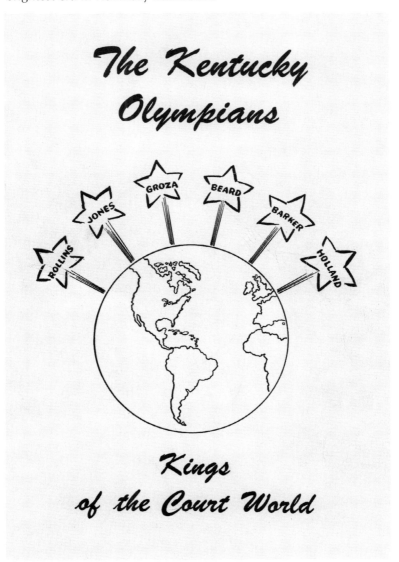

One Damn Great Basketball Team

In March 1950, Adolph Rupp was mad as hell.

His Wildcats were the defending national champions. They had won the Sugar Bowl Championship and the SEC Tournament. The Cats were ranked third in the nation. When the NCAA Tournament field was announced, Kentucky's name was not on the invitation list.

The country was divided into eight regions in those days and each region sent a team to the NCAA Tournament. The Selection Committee had a difficult time picking a team from Region 3 but Rupp was confident his team would be chosen over the other contender, North Carolina State. To Rupp's surprise, North Carolina State received the nod. Rupp made no secret of his disappointment and apparently the Selection Committee got the point. The next year, the field was expanded from eight teams to 16 with 10 conference champions and six independents comprising the field. Whether it was Rupp's protestations or not, it really made the NCAA Tournament a national event and harpooned the NIT, which had enjoyed at least equal prominence with the NCAA.

Everything was coming up roses for the Wildcats during the 1950-51 season. Memorial Coliseum had been completed and it was the most elegant arena on any college campus in the country. Seating capacity was 11,500 and several people had already

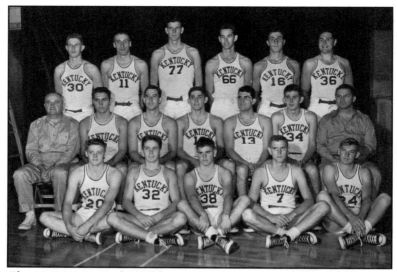

The 1950-51 Kentucky Wildcats. Front Row (L-R): Lindle Castle, Lucian Whitaker, Bobby Watson, Guy Strong, T. Riddle. Second Row: Head Coach Adolph Rupp, Cliff Hagan, C.M. Newton, Walt Hirsch, Paul Lansaw, Dwight Price, Asst. Coach Harry Lancaster. Back Row: Frank Ramsey, Shelby Linville, Bill Spivey, Roger Layne, Lou Tsioropoulos, Read Morgan.

branded it a "white elephant." Memorial Coliseum was built in dedication to Kentuckians who had lost their lives during World War II. The Coliseum was not just for basketball but was designed for concerts and lectures. Once, when the basketball team was displaced in order to prepare for a piano recital, Rupp was heard to grumble that if the maestro missed a note, nobody would know. On the other hand, if one of his players missed a key shot, everybody in the Coliseum would know.

The Wildcats not only had a grand new house but they were stocked with some fine basketball players. The only senior on the team was Walt Hirsch, who was also the final holdover from the "Fabulous Five." Hirsch would be permitted to play the entire regular-season but because he had played varsity ball as a freshman, he would not be eligible for tournament play. Hirsch, 6-4, was a very talented forward and a returning starter from the previous season. Kentucky was a junior-dominated team, led by the Wildcats' first seven-footer, Bill Spivey.

Rupp had read about Spivey in an Atlanta newspaper and invited the Warner Robins, Georgia, player to Lexington for a tryout. Rupp was not overly impressed with the seven-footer but he could not ignore the height factor and the way Spivey could run the floor. He asked Spivey to check in during the summer prior to his freshman year and Rupp put him under the wing of his trusted assistant, Harry Lancaster. Lancaster told me that Spivey was seven feet tall but weighed a skinny 165 pounds when he arrived at UK. Rupp had told Lancaster to not only work on Spivey's basketball skills but to try and get some weight on his thin frame. Rupp was in Europe that summer coaching the Olympic team and every two weeks, Harry would send Rupp a cable about Spivey's weight.

"When I finally sent the cable that Bill's weight had reached 185," Lancaster said, "the Baron sent his first cable back. It read, 'I know Spivey can eat, but can he play basketball?'" Spivey was a great basketball player by the time he reached his junior year.

On Spivey's freshman team, in 1949, there were 20 players on the squad. Bobby Watson was a 5-10 star from Owensboro, who Lancaster had asked to walk-on and try for a scholarship later. Bobby had been offered a partial scholarship at Alabama and caught the train to Tuscaloosa, Alabama, to check into the offer. When the coach did not show for almost two days, Watson caught the train back to Lexington and became a Wildcat.

That 1948-49 freshman team obtained great experience by scrimmaging against the "Fabulous Five" but when the season was complete, Rupp looked over the 20-man squad and selected only four players to join the varsity team for the next season: Spivey, Watson, Lucian "Skippy" Whitaker and C.M. Newton. They were battle-hardened juniors for the 1950-51 campaign.

Another junior was Shelby Linville, a 6-5 forward who had transferred from a junior college. Linville was a good shooter and rugged rebounder who brought great help to the Wildcats.

By the time the 1950-51 season rolled around, Rupp had decided on Spivey at center, Hirsch and Linville at the forwards. Watson and Whitaker would share one of the guard positions and at the other guard was a sophomore moving up from the freshman team, Frank Ramsey.

Frank was a gifted 6-3 player from Madisonville, Kentucky, who was hotly recruited by the Wildcats. He had been joined on the Kentucky freshman team for the second semester by Cliff Hagan from Owensboro, Kentucky, a mid-year high school graduate. The two later would be named All-Americans and inducted into the Basketball Hall of Fame. Despite living in towns in close proximity, they played against each other only once during their high school careers.

"Our junior year in high school," Ramsey said, "Owensboro Senior beat us something like 68-34. They doubled the score on us," he laughed.

During their high school senior years, Ramsey's team was eliminated in the Kentucky State Tournament and he accompanied the Wildcats to New York for the NCAA Tournament. Hagan's team won the State Championship for the 1949 season, as Cliff scored a record 49 points in the final game. Hagan left for New York a few days later and he and Ramsey took in the sights of the Big Apple as UK's guests.

Ramsey started the first game he was eligible during his sophomore year, but he was surprised to be starting as a guard. He had played center in high school and as a freshman at Kentucky he played both forward and center.

"I didn't play a second at guard," Frank said. When he reported for practice the next season, Frank told me, "Coach Rupp just said, 'You're a guard.'"

The first game ever played in Memorial Coliseum was on December 1, 1950 against West Texas State. It was a blowout with Kentucky winning, 73-43. The dedication game was a week later with UK whipping Purdue, 70-52. The Cats went on the road to de-

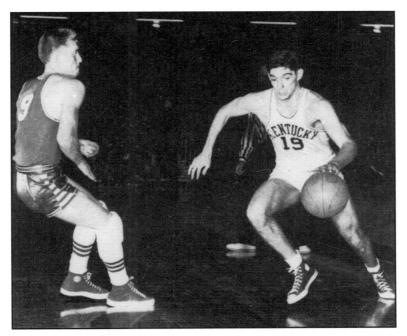

Walt Hirsch dribbles toward a Kansas defender during a highly anticipated game which pitted UK coach Adolph Rupp against his mentor, Phog Allen.

feat Xavier and returned home for an easy win over Florida. Then came a long awaited game with Kansas.

Fans had been anticipating the Kentucky-Kansas game even before the season began. The game was billed as the battle of the two best centers in college basketball, Bill Spivey of Kentucky and Clyde Lovelette of Kansas. The game also featured the first meeting between the winningest coach in college basketball, Phog Allen of Kansas, and his most famous pupil, Kentucky's Adolph Rupp.

Rupp was so nervous about playing against his former coach that he sent Harry Lancaster to scout Kansas during games in Philadelphia and New York. It was very rare to scout an opponent twice in those days but Rupp was very intent on winning. Lancaster's report suggested that the game would be decided by which center had a

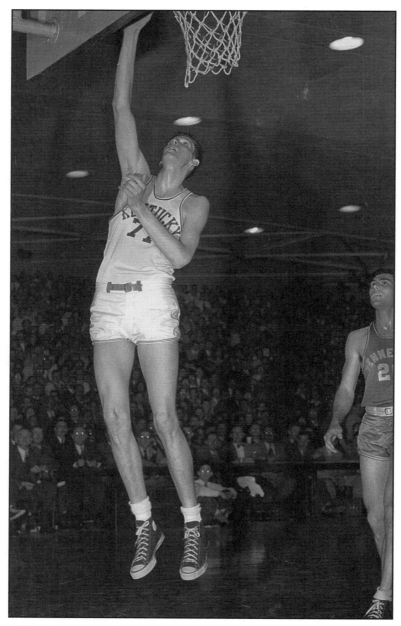

Bill Spivey, UK's first seven-footer, dominated college basketball and was the 1951 college Player of the Year.

better game. Lancaster also brought back all the papers from the two eastern cities, especially those articles that heaped praise on the great play of Lovelette. Each day he pasted several of them on Spivey's locker and each day Spivey ripped them down. Lancaster's supply was ample and he continued to put up new clippings each day. Just before the Wildcats left the dressing room to face Kansas, Rupp turned to Spivey and said, "Spivey, you can be the All-American center or you can let Lovelette be the All-American center. It's up to you." Spivey was up to the challenge.

Kentucky dominated right from the tipoff and Spivey turned in a whale of a game. Bobby Watson remembered that Spivey reached around Lovelette and deflected a pass, grabbed the loose ball and raced to the other end of the court for a tremendous dunk. "Nobody dunked in those days," Watson said. "That just brought the house down."

Lovelette fouled out with more than 13 minutes to play and Rupp immediately pulled Spivey from the lineup explaining later that he wanted the two centers to have exactly the same playing time. Spivey totally dominated the Kansas center, outscoring Lovelette 22-10 and Kentucky crushed the Jayhawks, 68-39.

The Cats went on the road to defeat St. John's, then lost for the first and only time during the regular season to St. Louis in the Sugar Bowl Tournament, 43-42 in overtime. Three days later, also in New Orleans, Paul "Bear" Bryant led the Kentucky football team to perhaps its greatest victory ever, defeating Oklahoma in the Sugar Bowl, 13-7. It was a tremendous upset as the Cats stopped Oklahoma's 47-game winning streak.

The Kentucky basketball team sailed on through the regular season, defeating Vanderbilt by 32 points to close out the campaign.

By winning the regular season SEC Championship, the Cats had qualified for the NCAA Tournament. This was the first time the regular season champion received an automatic bid to the big dance.

In the SEC Tournament in Louisville, the Cats breezed past Mississippi State, Auburn and Georgia Tech to advance to the final against Vanderbilt, a team it had trounced twice during the regular season. Vandy pulled a shocker and upset the Cats, 61-57.

"It was just one of those nights where nothing went right," Ramsey recalled. "We just stood around and Vandy played a good game."

Bobby Watson added, "We knew we were already in the NCAA and I think that had some effect. Nobody had a decent game for us."

A sportswriter described the Vandy win as the night "The calf slaughtered the butcher."

Perhaps it had become too easy for the Cats and, as it often happens, they moved to tournament play with a new focus and the resolve not to take any opponent too lightly.

Kentucky was paired against Louisville in Raleigh, North Carolina, in the first round of the NCAA Tournament. Coach Rupp was not pleased with the pairing but he had more serious things to be concerned about. He was in poor health. He had an eye infection and wore a patch over the eye. He had one leg in a cast.

Hirsch had played out his eligibility because he had been allowed to play with the varsity as a freshman. Now in his fourth season, he would not be permitted to play in the NCAA Tournament. Hagan took his place in the starting lineup. Hagan had become eligible for the varsity in mid-season and had been playing excellent basketball. Many thought his moving into the starting lineup actually made the Cats stronger.

"Hirsch was a good ball player but he was not the player Cliff was," Watson told me. "Without a doubt we were stronger with Cliff in the starting lineup."

The starters were now Linville and Hagan at the forwards, Spivey at center, and Ramsey and Watson at the guards. But the Cats still had a talented and deep bench. Coach Rupp could call on Whitaker, Newton, Guy Strong and Lou Tsioropoulos.

Louisville had a fine team that year and Kentucky trailed much of the game. Whitaker came off the bench in the second half and sparked the Cats to a 79-68 victory. Kentucky moved on to New

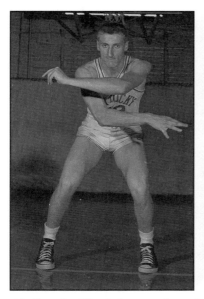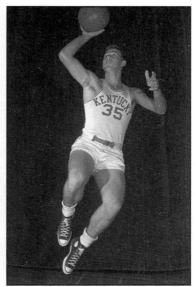

Shelby Linville (left) transferred to UK and became the Wildcats' second-leading scorer during the 1950-51 season, while C.M. Newton was a valuable contributor off the bench.

York for the East Regional where the Wildcats faced St. John's.

Kentucky had won a rather close decision over the Redmen in New York earlier in the season and expected another tough game. St. John's, with Al McGuire in the lineup, had set its game plan on holding down Spivey. It worked to some degree as Spivey was held to 12 points, about seven below his average, but Ramsey had a big game with 13 points and 12 rebounds and Watson added 12 points for the Wildcats as they won comfortably, 59-43. Next up for the Wildcats was a strong Illinois team.

Illinois was led by its captain, Don Sunderlage, who was having an awesome tournament. He scored 25 points as the Illini defeated Columbia, 79-71, halting the Lions' winning streak at 31 games. Sunderlage scored 21 points as Illinois romped past a strong North Carolina State team, 84-70. Kentucky knew it would not be a walk in the park against the Big Ten Champions.

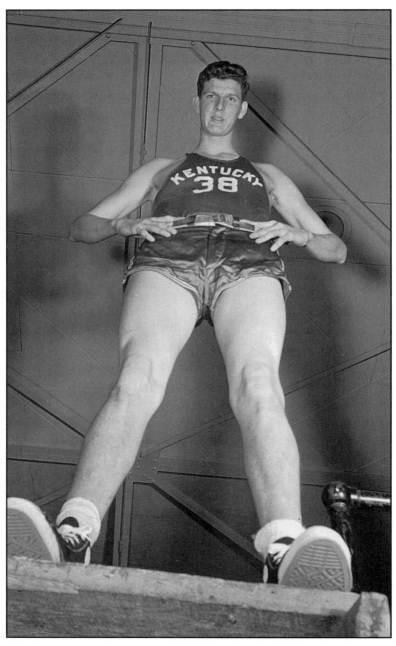

Bill Spivey was the most intimidating player of his era.

These two heavyweights came out slugging, but by the end of the first half Illinois held the advantage, 39-32. Spivey had an extraordinary game with 28 points and 16 rebounds, but when it got down to the nitty-gritty, he was on the bench with five fouls. Two of his teammates had also fouled out, Hagan and Whitaker. Linville picked up the slack late and actually scored the winning basket. Newton made a steal and fed the ball to Linville who hit the game-winner with 12 seconds remaining and the Cats advanced to the championship game with a 76-74 squeaker over Illinois.

The Kentucky Wildcats would represent the East Region against the Kansas State Wildcats from the West Region in Minneapolis.

The championship game was scheduled for March 27, 1951, at Williams Arena on the campus of the University of Minnesota. Ramsey said it was the first time he ever saw a portable floor put down on top of dirt. Planks were placed on top of the dirt from the dressing room all the way to the floor. The players had to wipe their sneakers on towels to keep from slipping on the hardwood. Still, the arena in Minneapolis was spacious and a packed house of 15,428 turned out for the title game.

Kansas State came into the game with an awesome reputation. Coach Jack Gardner had traveled all over the country to bring in the best talent he had ever assembled. He prided himself on the great balance the team from Manhattan, Kansas, put on the court. He would often platoon his players, sending in an entire new unit at a time. Gardner was a fanatic about milk. He kept several bottles under his bench and would consume up to a gallon of the good white stuff during a game. The Kansas State brand of Wildcats had beaten some of the best teams in the country and totally destroyed one of them, Oklahoma A&M, in the finals of the West Regional in Kansas City, 68-44.

The Oklahoma A&M coach, Henry Iba, and Rupp were the two giants of college coaching, but they were also fast friends. They served on some committees together and each always held the other in high regard. Iba, who was attending the finals in Minneapolis, told

Rupp that Kansas State was the best team in basketball history and that there was no way Kentucky could win. Rupp snorted, "The hell with that. We've got to find some way to beat them."

Rupp wasn't just worried about Kansas State. His All-American, Bill Spivey, was suffering from a heavy cold. Cliff Hagan, who had played magnificently in the tournament, had the flu and was running a fever. Rupp moved Ramsey to forward, with Watson and Whitaker playing the guard positions. Hagan, under doctors orders, would be held out of the game. Rupp himself might have been in the worst condition of them all. He was still wearing that big eye patch and had a big steel and leather brace on his leg. He had been too ill to attend the team's pre-game meeting and arrived at the arena just in time for the game. He told his players just before they left the locker room, "I'm in misery but don't worry about me. Just go out there and play your game."

Perhaps it was the effect of the cold, but Spivey's performance in the first half was lethargic and he was completely outplayed by Lew Hitch of Kansas State. The Big Seven Conference Champions had Kentucky down by two points at the intermission, 29-27.

As if Rupp's ailments didn't give him enough pain, the play of his basketball team inflicted even more misery. He read them the riot act in the dressing room.

"Coach Rupp and Coach Lancaster had a few choice words for us at the half," Ramsey recalled. "I remember exactly what they said, but you sure couldn't print it."

Rupp told Hagan, sick or not, he was going to start the second half and Ramsey would go back to his regular guard position. The team went out to play the final 20 minutes of the championship game.

Whatever he said to Spivey seemed to build a fire under the seven-footer. He was brilliant in the second half and finished the game with 22 points and 21 rebounds. Hagan was the catalyst who elevated the Cats to victory. He scored 10 points and grabbed some key rebounds. The second half belonged to Kentucky and the Cats won it going away, 68-58. Gardner liked to point out the overall balance of Kansas State but Kentucky proved to have great balance too. Ramsey and Whitaker scored nine points apiece and Watson and Linville each turned in an eight-point performance in the championship game.

At breakfast the next morning, Iba accused Rupp of running a delay game against Kansas State. Rupp denied it but Lancaster told me Kentucky did indeed slow it down in the last part of the game. Rupp felt so bad during the game that he turned UK's controls over to Lancaster and Harry felt that the Kentucky team was in such poor shape physically, with Spivey and Hagan ailing, that it would be best to go for only easy shots. Lancaster said the team had practiced the delay but just hadn't needed it until the Kansas State game.

It was the third time in four years that Kentucky had won the NCAA Championship and it appeared there was no end in sight for the Wildcats. Coach Rupp had everybody returning from that championship team for the next season including the college Player of the Year, Spivey. At least that's what he thought in late March 1951. Six months later, Kentucky's hopes came crashing down. The point-shaving scandal in college basketball raised its ugly head and UK was one of the schools being investigated. Coach Rupp said they couldn't touch his players "with a 10-foot pole," but that turned out to be false. Some of the players on the "Fabulous Five" were implicated, but they were long gone from the university. But then, UK officials informed Rupp that Spivey was being investigated and ordered the Kentucky coach not to play the seven-footer next season. Later, a jury in New York voted 9-3 for Spivey's acquittal but, unfortunately, the big fellow's basketball days at Kentucky were over.

I have always felt that the 1951 team at Kentucky was the forgotten team among the six NCAA Championship teams. I don't know if it was overshadowed by the investigation and later punishment of the school for the player's involvement in the point-shaving scandal, but for some reason that team just never received the notoriety of the other five champions. Bobby Watson made a case for his team when we discussed my beliefs.

"I think that team is overlooked but it was a VERY good team," he said. "Cliff and Frank were both on that team and they're in the Hall of Fame now. Spivey was an All-American on that team and was the best player in the country that year."

That was an excellent college basketball team. It had size, quickness and played great defense. It was a tremendous rebounding team and despite Spivey's scoring accomplishments, there was great balance on the club. An opponent couldn't key on any one player and hope to stop the Wildcats.

Kentucky played some of the best teams in the country that season and lost only twice — a one-point overtime decision to St. Louis and a four-point loss to Vanderbilt in the SEC Tournament — by a total of five points. Their record at the end of the year was a brilliant 32-2 and that, of course, included the Wildcats' third NCAA Championship trophy.

In his book, written in 1979, Harry Lancaster wrote "Looking back through the years, I never felt that team got the credit it deserved. Perhaps it was because it was never branded with a catchy label like the 'Fabulous Five,' or the 'Fiddlin' Five,' or 'Rupp's Runts,' but for anybody who ever saw that 1951 team play, it was one damn great basketball team."

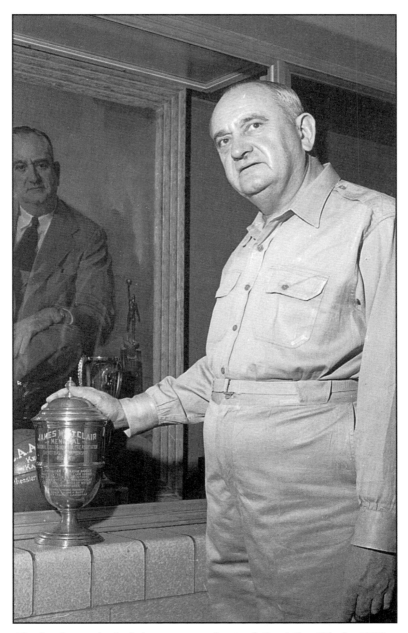

Having been denied the opportunity to defend the title in 1950,
Rupp especially relished Kentucky's 1951 NCAA Championship.

They Sure Could Fiddle

No player was considered good enough to be named to the All-Conference team, but together they won the national championship. The 1957-58 team gave Adolph Rupp his fourth NCAA Championship at Kentucky.

The glory years of the Fabulous Five and the Hagan-Ramsey eras were gone. There were mutterings that Rupp had lost it and I doubt that any team ever gave him as much satisfaction as that 1958 team did. It came as such a surprise.

He didn't sound all that confident as he gathered the players for the start of that season.

"We're all fiddlers, that's all," he said. "They're pretty good fiddlers ... be right entertaining at a barn dance. But I'll tell you, you need violinists to play at Carnegie Hall. We don't have any violinists."

Rupp's assessment of his players earned them their nickname, the "Fiddlin' Five." He had also correctly labeled the schedule a "Carnegie Hall" caliber worksheet.

Kentucky had a veteran starting lineup returning with four seniors and a junior. Vernon Hatton, Ed Beck and John Crigler had all come to the university together. Adrian Smith, the other senior, had come from the junior college ranks and was in his second year with the Wildcats.

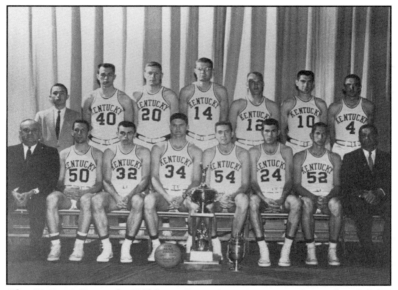

The 1957-58 Kentucky Wildcats. Front Row (L-R): Head Coach Adolph Rupp, Adrian Smith, John Crigler, Ed Beck, Don Mills, Johnny Cox, Vernon Hatton, Asst. Coach Harry Lancaster. Back Row: Mgr. Jay Atkerson, Earl Adkins, Billy Smith, Phil Johnson, Bill Cassady, Lincoln Collinsworth, Harold Ross.

Hatton, a 6-3 guard, was the team captain. Vernon had been a star at Lafayette High School in Lexington under a former UK star, Ralph Carlisle. Hatton was an excellent shooter and had tremendous basketball savvy. He didn't have blinding speed but he could maneuver well among defenders and could score on either his jump shot or by driving toward the basket. Hatton's best attribute was that he was a winner. Harry Lancaster, Rupp's assistant for 26 years, said of Hatton, "He had great confidence in himself and he's the man you wanted to have the ball when it got down to the nitty gritty." Hatton was one of the best clutch players to ever wear the blue and white.

Adrian "Odie" Smith was the other guard. Smith had been a standout high school player at Farmington, Kentucky, but at 5-10, 150-pounds, Rupp thought he might be too small to play for the Wildcats. "Odie" had an outstanding junior college career in Mississippi and after he averaged more than 27 points a game his second year, Coach Rupp was glad to welcome him as a Wildcat. Odie was probably a little intimidated by the other four starters for the 1957-58 season. Hatton said they called him in and told Smith to stop shooting the ball so much and to pass it more. Odie's star rose after he left UK and he had the most distinguished career in pro ball of all the "fiddlers."

Beck was a 6-7 center. The senior from Georgia had suffered a personal tragedy near the end of the preceding season when his wife, Billie, died of cancer. The other players rallied around Beck and they became a very close-knit team. Lancaster said the 1958 team was the closest of any UK team during his 26-year coaching stint. Beck was not much of a scorer in the legacy of other UK centers, but he was a great defensive player and rebounder. He was totally unselfish and his bone-jarring picks for Hatton and Johnny Cox were extremely instrumental in that team's success. Ed was one of the finest young men to ever wear a Kentucky uniform.

Crigler played one of the forward positions. He was only 6-3 and was not a renowned shooter from the outside, but John had a knack for driving to the basket. "Crig" was a hard-nosed defensive player but his strong suit was his hustle. John was playing at full speed every second he was on the court.

Cox, the other forward, was a 6-4 junior from Hazard, Kentucky. All four starters, with the exception of Beck, were Kentuckians and Johnny had been a huge high school star before joining the Wildcats. He was skinny as a snake and as tough as hickory. Other teams banged him around pretty good, but the tougher they tried to make it on Cox, the better he played. He was an outstanding outside shooter and had an accurate little hook-shot with either hand. A few years ago, I met the owner of the New York Yankees, George Steinbrenner, on the backstretch at Churchill Downs in Louisville. Jim Morgan, who had been a fine player at Louisville, was training some horses for Steinbrenner. At the time Jim told him

I had been broadcasting UK's games for a long time and Steinbrenner volunteered that Cox was the best shooter he ever saw. It turned out that Cox had played for the Cleveland Pipers, an industrial team that Steinbrenner owned. George was right on the money in describing Johnny's talent.

Hatton, Smith, Beck, Crigler and Cox were the starters on that 1958 NCAA Championship team.

The Season

The "barnyard fiddlers" got the campaign off to a good start with a win at home over Duke and a victory over Ohio State on the road. The Wildcats returned to Memorial Coliseum to take on the Temple Owls, and that turned out to be one of the most exciting games in Kentucky's storied history.

Hatton made a free throw with 49 seconds remaining in the game to tie the score at 65. Smith missed a desperation heave at the buzzer and the contest went to overtime. In the extra stanza, Kentucky seemed to be beaten when Temple's outstanding guard, Guy Rodgers, hit a 15-foot shot to push the Owls ahead by two points with only three seconds left. By the time Kentucky took a timeout, only one second blinked on the Coliseum scoreboard.

The crowd seemed to say, "Outta Here." I recall that scene as if it were yesterday. By the time that timeout was over, half the crowd had cleared the Coliseum to get a jump on the traffic for the trip home.

In the UK huddle, Rupp turned to Smith and said, "Smitty, you've got to try it again, but make it this time." Harry Lancaster said he could tell by the look on Hatton's face that Vernon wanted to take that last shot and he suggested to Rupp that they let Hatton take it. "I heard him say that," Hatton said. "Yeah Coach, let me take it."

The stage was set. One second to play. Kentucky had the ball at mid-court. Crigler would put it in play. Temple expected Kentucky to throw toward the basket and sagged its defense. Crigler passed

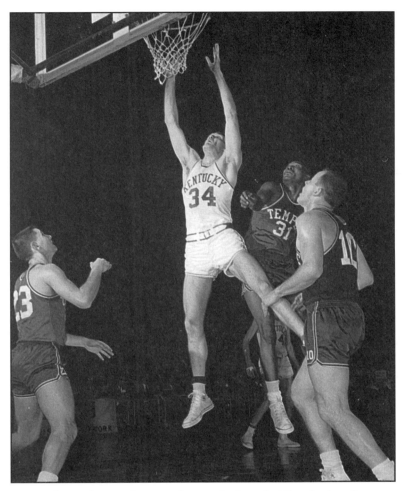

***Kentucky and Temple waged two glorious battles during the
1957-58 season.***

the ball in to Hatton and in one motion he let the long two-handed shot fly. Bingo. Nothing but net. The game was tied and moved
to a second overtime.

The distance of Hatton's shot has varied over the years, so I
went directly to Vernon for the answer. "It was 48 feet, 10 inches," he said.

The second overtime settled nothing as the score was dead-locked at 75. Kentucky finally prevailed at the end of the third overtime, 85-83. What I remember, thinking back, was that when I looked around during that last overtime, the crowd had gradual-ly moved back inside the Coliseum and the place was again packed when the game was over. Apparently, the fans had been lis-tening to the game on the radio when Hatton made his heroic shot and they came back in to watch the end. They couldn't have been disappointed.

The next day Hatton went by Rupp's office to ask if he could have the game ball from the Temple game. "Give you the game ball?" asked an incredulous Rupp. "Just because you scored two points from 47 feet with one second to go, you want me to give you the game ball? How would I explain that to the Athletics Board, giving away a $35 basketball?"

Hatton was furious. He was about to get up and storm out of the meeting when a big grin creased Rupp's face. He reached under the desk and pitched the ball to Vernon and said, "Congratulations, son." Coach Rupp told him, "Tell your grandchildren about it."

The "fiddlers" struggled on through the season and when they lost a one-point decision to Auburn in Birmingham, it marked their sixth loss of the season. The Cats went into Knoxville for the next game, the final contest of the season, having to beat Tennessee to gain the SEC Championship and the automatic bid to the NCAA Tournament. With Smith having a big game, the Cats defeated the Vols, 77-66.

Kentucky finished the regular-season with a 19-6 record, the Wildcats' worst mark since the 1940-41 season.

No team had ever won the NCAA Championship with six loss-es and the Wildcats were given little chance of fiddlin' their way to the title in 1958. The experts didn't count on two things: Kentucky would play the entire tournament within the boundaries of the Commonwealth and the Wildcats had saved their best basketball for the final four games of the year.

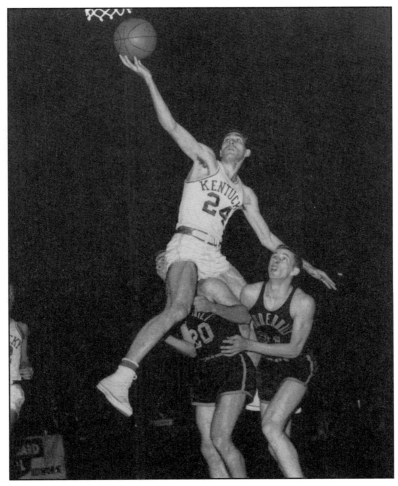

The tougher the play became, the better Johnny Cox performed.

It is a misnomer to call the 1958 team the "Fiddlin' Five." The team had tremendous depth even though Coach Rupp rarely used more than eight players in a game.

Most of them had come in together in the freshman class for the 1954-55 season. Earl Adkins had been a high school star from Ashland, Kentucky. Billy Ray Cassady was a high-scoring guard from Inez, Kentucky. Also included in that class were Lincoln

105

Collinsworth, Harold Ross and Bill Smith, along with the trio that would end up as starters four years later, Beck, Crigler and Hatton.

Freshmen were ineligible to play with the varsity in those days, so they played their own schedule. Lancaster coached the frosh. Hatton remembered that in a game against Sue Bennett Junior College, the Kentucky yearlings were leading 127-25 when a timeout was called. One of the players asked Lancaster what he wanted the team to run. Lancaster, for a change, was at a loss for words. "Frankly, I don't know," he said. "I was never leading by 102 points before."

Johnny Cox came to UK the next year and Smith transferred to UK the following year. Don Mills became a member of the "fiddlers" for the 1957-58 season and brought an important contribution to the Wildcats.

The Tournament

On March 14, 1958, Kentucky began the big dance on its home court in Memorial Coliseum in the Mideast Regional. With Cox pouring in 23 points, Kentucky had a surprisingly easy time with a good Miami of Ohio team to the tune of a 94-70 victory. The Wildcats had been impressive in their opening win but they were given next-to-no-chance the next night against a strong Notre Dame team that had beaten Big Ten champion Indiana in the other semifinal. Tom Hawkins, the gifted All-American for the Irish, had riddled the Hoosier defense for 31 points.

Coach Rupp realized he had to devise a plan to at least slow Hawkins down for the Cats to have any chance at winning. He decided that Beck would play directly behind Hawkins and that Smith would drop back and play in front of the Irish star. Kentucky would give up some outside shots to Notre Dame with this scheme but Rupp thought the gamble was worth it. Lancaster said that even though it was several years later that most people gave Rupp credit for playing a zone defense for the first time, his plan for Notre Dame certainly resembled a zone. "... we came awfully close to one that night. Smitty sat in Hawkins' lap all night and we held him to 15

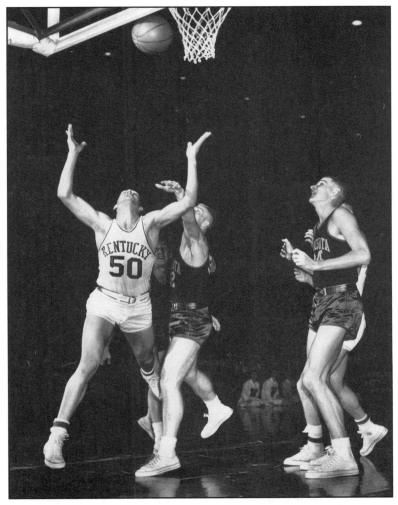

Originally, Rupp didn't believe Adrian "Odie" Smith could play for Kentucky. However, after Smith transferred to UK, he became an integral part of the Fiddlin' Five.

points." Rupp's plan worked to perfection as Kentucky demolished Notre Dame, 89-56. It would have been considered a monumental upset if Kentucky had emerged a one-point winner, but the Wildcats handed the Irish one of their worst defeats in history.

107

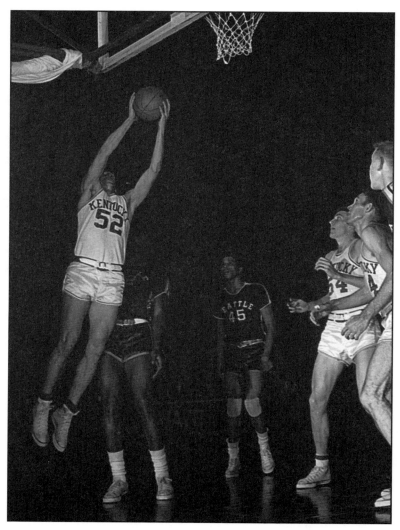

Vernon Hatton scored a game-high 30 points in the 1958 NCAA Championship game while ...

The Final Four

Kentucky had to travel only 80 miles for the Final Four, which was scheduled for Freedom Hall in Louisville. There, the Wildcats joined Kansas State, Seattle and their old friends, the Temple Owls.

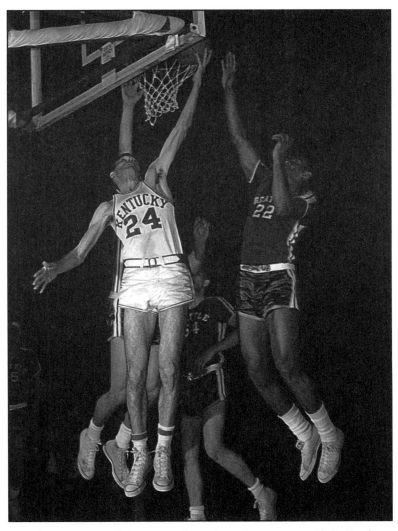

... Johnny Cox and Company kept Seattle superstar Elgin Baylor busy all night.

Freedom Hall might not have been Carnegie Hall, but in 1958 it was the largest, grandest basketball arena in America.

Kentucky faced Temple in the first semifinal. The Owls, since losing the triple-overtime game to Kentucky in Lexington, had lost

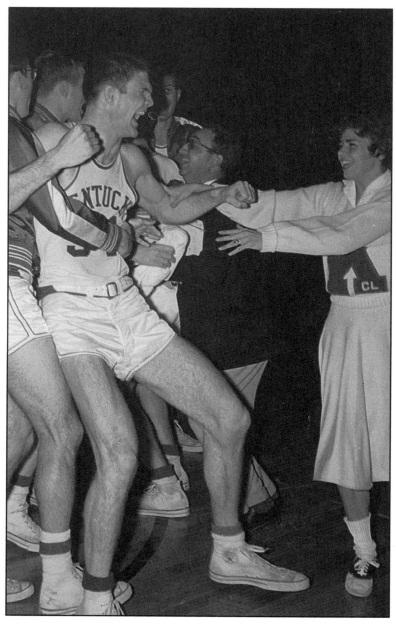

The Cats converge on UK center Ed Beck after the horn sounded, celebrating Kentucky's fourth NCAA title.

only to Cincinnati and the great Oscar Robertson to bring a sparkling 26-2 record into the game.

It was another barn-burner. With 24 seconds to play and Temple leading 60-59, Rupp signaled for a timeout. He set up a play for Hatton to take a shot from the outside, but Ed Beck made a suggestion. The Kentucky center told Rupp that the defensive center hadn't switched all night and that if Hatton would drive off Beck's screen, Vernon would be open. "All right," Rupp told the players, "forget what I told you and let's go with Beck's play."

Hatton put down his dribble and drove by Beck but as he neared the basket he found himself surrounded by Temple defenders. He drove past the basket for a reverse layup that pushed Kentucky into a 61-60 lead. There were 16 seconds left to play.

Lady luck smiled on the Cats as Temple's Bill "Pickles" Kennedy fumbled the ball out of bounds and Kentucky advanced to the championship game.

There were some who questioned Rupp for scoring with too much time left on the clock, but the winning coach grumbled, "Hell, you never get a basket too quick when you are one point behind with seconds to go." The criticism was foolish since Rupp had instructed his players to all go for the rebound in case Hatton missed the shot. He didn't and the Wildcats were set to play for the national title.

Rupp and the team dressed and sat in the stands to watch the second semifinal between Kansas State and Seattle. It was another intense battle with Seattle leading the favored Wildcats from Kansas State, 37-32, at the half. Rupp took the team back to the hotel during the intermission, leaving Lancaster and trusted scout Elmer "Baldy" Gilb to chart the game and make recommendations about winning against either opponent. Rupp was spared watching the slaughter. In one of the greatest performances I ever saw, Elgin Baylor put on a one-man clinic in the second half, blocking shots, firing behind-the-back passes and scoring at will. He personally embarrassed Kansas State as Seattle won 73-51. Baylor had 23

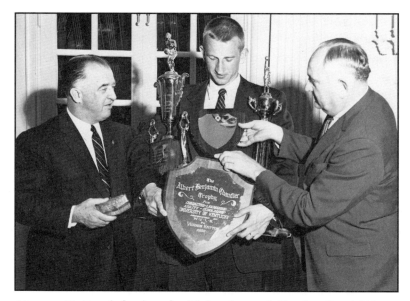

Vernon Hatton is besieged with hardware following the 1958 season, his last as a Wildcat. (Left: Kentucky Governor A.B. "Happy" Chandler; Right: Adolph Rupp.)

points and 22 rebounds. Lancaster and Gilb just looked at each other after the game and agreed they had no scouting report.

Lancaster carried the bad news back to Rupp at the Seelbach Hotel where the team was quartered. He told Rupp that Baylor had made monkeys out of Kansas State. "There's no way we can beat them," he told his boss.

It wasn't like Rupp or Lancaster to admit defeat, but when they met with the team at lunch the next day, their scouting report was so poor, the team felt it had next-to-no chance of winning. The coaches sent the team to bed to await the Seattle game later that evening.

If ever a coach was more pleased to see a total stranger on game day, it is shrouded in mystery. A knock at Coach Rupp's hotel room door produced an obscure coach from Idaho, John Grayson, who said he had come to tell Rupp how to beat Seattle.

"To beat Seattle," Grayson told Rupp, "the thing is you must convince your kids that they can't stand there and watch Baylor play. He mesmerizes them." Grayson then showed Rupp and Lancaster a film he had brought with him, pointing out that Baylor had a difficult time guarding a player who would drive on him. He told the Kentucky coaches that if they could get Baylor in foul trouble they could defeat Seattle.

Rupp was really excited with the report Grayson had given him. "Wake these kids 30 minutes early," he told Lancaster. "We'll give them this new scouting report."

While Lancaster thought Grayson's scouting report was vital, he thought the fact that he and Rupp finally had come up with a scouting report meant just as much. He said he could see in the players' eyes that they were gaining confidence during the scouting report. "Now, you could see them getting fired up," he said. "It was go."

When I walked into Freedom Hall that night of March 22, 1958, I was among those who thought Seattle might be too much for the Cats. I think, to this day, that Elgin Baylor was one of the best I saw play in all my years behind the play-by-play microphone. I felt that Kentucky might have used up its miracles the night before against Temple. Yes, they played the semifinals and the final on successive nights in those days. I've always been a stickler for preparation and I worked into the wee hours of the next morning to get ready for the Kentucky-Seattle game. I arrived at Freedom Hall early on game day and went directly to the press room where the statistics had been updated and continued to work on the game. As game time approached, and the partisan Kentucky crowd started coming in, I began to feel the Cats had a real shot at Seattle. I didn't know about Grayson's visit at that time but I was feeling more confident as we approached the tip-off.

Rupp was certain that Baylor would guard Beck, the only starter who was not averaging in double figures. To Coach Rupp's delight, Baylor lined up defensively on Crigler and Rupp ordered his senior forward to drive and drive on the Seattle star. Apparently Seattle Coach John Castellani had scouted Kentucky's squeaker over Tem-

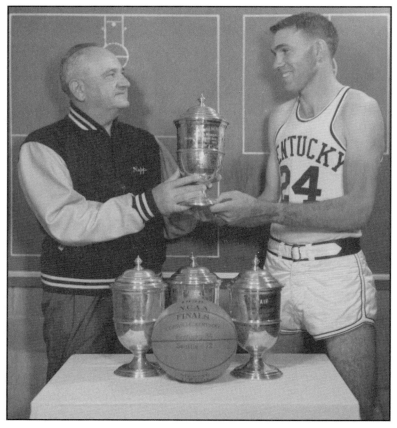

Adolph Rupp and Johnny Cox admire Kentucky's fourth NCAA Championship trophy.

ple the night before and noticed that Crigler had had a poor shooting performance, going 3 of 11. Kentucky moved the ball to Crigler over and over and he set sail for the basket, as Baylor picked up three early fouls. Castellani then switched his star to guard Beck and Don Mills. Rupp told Hatton to drive off Beck's screens and force Baylor to either let him go or risk picking up a fourth foul. Vernon lit it up. After Baylor picked up his fourth foul trying to block a Mills hook shot, Seattle dropped back into a zone and Johnny Cox poured it in from long range. Although Baylor had 25 points and 19 rebounds, Kentucky rolled to a surprisingly easy win, 84-72, to give Rupp his fourth and last NCAA Championship. Hatton scored 30 points and Cox added 24 for the Wildcats.

"They weren't the greatest basketball players in the world," Rupp would say later. "All they could do was win." He called them the "Fiddlin' Five" and Rupp was sticking with it. "These boys are still just a bunch of barnyard fiddlers, but they sure can fiddle!"

The Season of No Celebration

Wildcat fans had waited impatiently for two decades. Not since Kentucky won the 1958 NCAA Championship had the Cats reached the charmed circle. Oh, there had been close calls and near misses, but no NCAA titles until the Wildcats won UK's fifth championship in 1978.

Coach Rupp had taken the Wildcats to the championship game in 1966, but Kentucky was upset by Texas Western. In 1972, at the age of 70, Rupp went reluctantly into retirement and one of his former players and assistants, Joe B. Hall, took over the Wildcat fortunes.

In 1975, Joe B. led the Cats all the way to the NCAA Tournament final game before losing to UCLA in John Wooden's last game as a coach. The freshmen that year played an important role and would be the nucleus at Kentucky for the next three years.

The next season, Hall's youthful Cats started the year at 10-10, but ran off 10 straight victories, including the NIT Championship.

"That team was the most fun to coach of any team I had at Kentucky," Hall said. Hall liked the scrappy way the team played and was pleased by its improvement as the season went along.

That was the last team to play in Memorial Coliseum. The Cats started the next campaign in Rupp Arena.

That season, the 1976-77 year, Kentucky put together a fancy

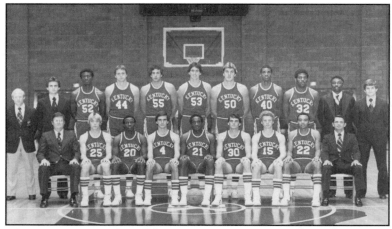

The 1977-78 Kentucky Wildcats. Front Row (L-R): Head Coach Joe B. Hall, Jay Shidler, Dwane Casey, Kyle Macy, Jack Givens, Tim Stephens, Chris Gettelfinger, Truman Claytor, Asst. Coach Dickie Parsons. Back Row: Asst. Trainer Walt McCombs, Mgr. Don Sullivan, LaVon Williams, Scott Courts, Mike Phillips, Rick Robey, Chuck Aleksinas, Fred Cowan, James Lee, Asst. Coach Leonard Hamilton, Asst. Coach Joe Dean.

26-4 record that ended with a seven-point loss to North Carolina in the East Regional of the NCAA Tournament.

Hall thought his 1977-78 team would be his best yet.

"We had almost the same team returning," Hall said. "Our only major loss was Larry Johnson, one of the best defensive guards we ever had. We had Kyle Macy coming in and I knew he would bring a lot to the team."

Macy had sat out the previous season after transferring from Purdue. He had studied film of the Kentucky team during the summer and, Hall said, "Macy could run our whole offense on the first day of practice. That impressed me. I had never seen a player come in for his first practice with us and know all the plays. He had a full year to practice with us and I knew he would be a big help that season."

A pair of 6-10 bookends, Rick Robey and Mike Phillips, gave Kentucky the strong inside game. Macy would team up with Truman Claytor at guard. Jack Givens would play the small forward.

Hall's assistant, Jim Hatfield, was the first to take a look at Robey, and he liked what he saw. When Joe B. went to New Orleans to scout the high school star, he spotted Notre Dame's Digger Phelps in the audience. Phelps later decided Robey was too slow for the system the Irish were using.

"I absolutely loved him," Hall told me. "I never saw a guy his size play with such intensity. He wasn't afraid to go after a loose ball and to slide on his belly."

Robey always played with great intensity at Kentucky and he made the starting lineup as a freshman.

When Hall began recruiting Phillips, he knew the big guy could score. Mike had broken Jerry Lucas' Ohio high school scoring records. Hall's biggest concern about Phillips was that he didn't run the court very well. At Kentucky, Phillips developed better technique in his running style and became a fine player. Mike had the heart of a lion. He never backed away from anything.

Phillips was listed as the center and Robey at forward, but they were interchangeable in those two positions. As far as I know, they were the original "Twin Towers" in basketball.

The other starting forward on that team was Givens. Jack was only 6-4 and played more out on the court. They called him "Goose," but he was like a ballet dancer. He was as smooth as silk and was deadly accurate with that left hand shot. Givens had been an outstanding player at Bryan Station High School in Lexington, and had been at the top of the UK recruiting list for several years.

Phillips, Robey and Givens were seniors on that 1977-78 starting team and all had played extensively since their freshman season.

Claytor, a junior, started at one of the guard positions. Kentucky had become involved late in the recruiting race on Truman. Hall was holding the scholarship for Kyle Macy, a high school star from Peru, Indiana, but Macy was slow to commit and Hall knew that Purdue was very much in the picture. With Leonard Hamilton, one of Hall's assistants, leading the charge, Claytor became a Wildcat. The Toledo, Ohio, native was very quick and could really play defense. He was a little streaky in shooting from the outside but when

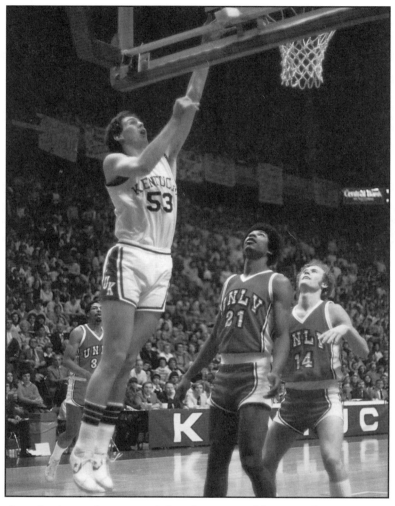

As a freshman in 1975, Rick Robey was a big part of UK's NCAA Tournament runner-up team. In 1978, he was determined to win the national championship.

Claytor had his eye, he could fill it up from long range.

Ironically, the other starting guard on that team was Macy. After transferring from Purdue and sitting out a year, the 6-3 sophomore proved to be the missing part of the puzzle. He was a deadly marksman from long range and brought great intelligence and leadership to the team.

The fourth senior on the team was 6-5, 230-pound James Lee out of Henry Clay High School in Lexington. Lee and Givens had both been stars in high school but adversaries at the same time. James was as strong as a bull. He had such a menacing countenance that women wanted to get their children out of harm's way when Lee was around. Macy said that players on other teams were always asking him if James was as mean as he looked out there on the floor. Macy said, "James was just the opposite. He would do anything in the world for you and didn't have a mean bone in his body. James was a big cut-up."

In my mind, James Lee was absolutely the best sixth man in college basketball that season. Even though Lee came in from the bench, Hall never considered him a sub.

"James was really a starter. We actually started Phillips and Robey, knowing that one of them would probably get in foul trouble. James was that catalyst that would come in fresh, after we had taken a little edge off the opponent, and he would really pick us up."

Lee wasn't the only support Hall could rely upon coming off the bench. Jay Shidler was, from time to time, a starter at one of the guard spots and could shoot the lights out. Also ready for duty were LaVon Williams, Dwane Casey, Freddie Cowan, Tim Stephens and others. Kentucky had a deep and talented support cast.

The 1977-78 season got off to a rocky start. On "Press Day," the day before the beginning of practice, Shidler showed up on crutches. He was expected to be a strong candidate for a starting job but had broken his foot.

The words, "get a wall," struck terror in the hearts of the UK players. It was Hall's form of punishment for missing breakfast, missing a class, missing curfew or some other team rule violation. To "get a wall," a player had to run from the playing floor to the top of Memorial Coliseum. He then would touch the wall and run back to the playing floor.

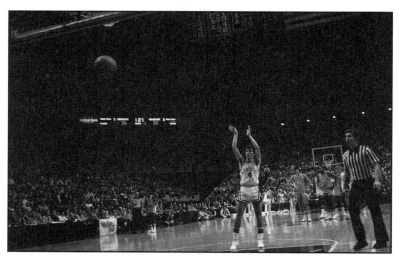

After transferring from Purdue, Kyle Macy spent a season on the sidelines, learning the Kentucky system inside and out.

On the last day of October, Hall showed up with a list of players' names. They had breached the rules and he ordered them to run 25 walls. Lee refused and walked out of practice. He didn't return for two days, but he came back, ran his walls and rejoined the team.

In the preseason, the Wildcats defeated the Soviet Union Olympic Team, 109-75. Alexander Gomelsky, the feisty little coach of the visitors, in his broken English said, "Best team I ever look." The Cats were off to a roaring start.

Two games during the season readily come to mind. The first was Kentucky's initial road game of the campaign. The Cats were playing Coach Rupp's alma mater, Kansas, and it was a close game in jam-packed Allen Fieldhouse. The date was December 10, 1977. Kentucky won the game, but it was to become a sad evening. As we got back to the motel after the game, we learned that Coach Rupp had died. We all knew he was very sick and was not likely to recover, but to lose the man who had meant so much to Kentucky — and to me — left me with a heavy heart.

Kentucky's first loss of the campaign came at Alabama, 15 games into the season. C.M. Newton's fine team defeated the Cats, 78-62. But it was the very next road trip by the Wildcats that is even more vivid in my memory. It was perhaps the worst performance of the season for Kentucky as it lost in overtime to LSU, 95-94. To add to the humiliation, all five LSU starters had fouled out during regulation play and the Bayou Bengals won with their subs. Hall was seething after the game. Some of Kentucky's best teams had nicknames like the "Fabulous Five" and the "Fiddlin' Five," but on our postgame radio program from Baton Rouge, Louisiana, Hall made the suggestion to his audience that this team should be called the "Foldin' Five."

The team moved on to Oxford, Mississippi, and a date with the Ole Miss Rebels. Hall was still visibly angry. Every time a player made any kind of mistake, Hall jerked him from the lineup. He made 17 substitutions in the first half alone. It was not a thing of beauty, but Kentucky won and apparently Hall had the players' attention. They waltzed through the remainder of the schedule and claimed another SEC Championship.

Hall had been under intense pressure since taking over the head coaching position from the legendary Rupp. After Wooden announced his decision to retire following the Kentucky game in the NCAA finals in 1975, Hall joked that he should get the UCLA job since he was the only coach in the world experienced at following a legend. Joe B. might have meant it as a joke, but there was a lot of truth in the comment. Now, to get the monkey off his back, Hall desperately needed to win the NCAA Championship.

The Wildcats' quest for the title began in Knoxville, Tennessee, against Hugh Durham's Florida State team. Hall felt his Wildcats could beat Florida State.

"I felt we just had a better team," he said.

The Seminoles shocked Kentucky right out of the gate. Florida State zipped to a 10-point lead in the first half and still led by seven at the intermission, 39-32.

"They were getting out on the fast break for easy baskets," Hall said. "We were not getting back on defense. We were playing very lethargic."

Joe B. read the riot act to his players during the session in the dressing room. He told them they were not giving him an honest effort and that he was going to go with the players in the second half who would give him an all-out effort. He announced that Macy and Phillips were the only starters who would begin the second half. He was going with Casey, Cowan and Williams while the other starters could take a seat on the bench. It was a daring and bold gamble, so bold some believed, that it could have cost Hall his job had it not been successful.

As the team left the dressing room for the second half, Hall turned to his top aide, Dick Parsons, and said, "If this doesn't work, we're getting out of town. We're not even going back to Lexington. We may never be able to go back."

Hall's makeshift team acquitted itself well, actually cutting two points off Florida State's lead. Phillips was playing very well. Hall said, "He played perhaps his finest half of basketball in his life."

When Hall put the starters back in, they blew Florida State away and eased out to an 85-76 win. Kyle Macy said, "We had been lucky. We had won on a bad day."

Kentucky had dodged the bullet. Joe B.'s gamble had paid off. He had thrown a seven.

Kentucky moved north to Dayton, Ohio, for the Mideast Regional to face Miami of Ohio, a surprise winner over Marquette in the first round.

Kentucky came out on fire in the first half. Claytor took five shots and made them all. Phillips matched him with 10 points in the first half as Kentucky breezed to an easy lead, 46-30. The Cats kept up their fine play in the second half as Phillips had his day in the sun to lead Kentucky with 24 points. Four of his teammates also scored in double figures. Kentucky coasted to an easy win, 91-69.

The Cats expected a war with Michigan State in the Mideast Regional final and the Spartans delivered. State's 2-3 zone sealed off

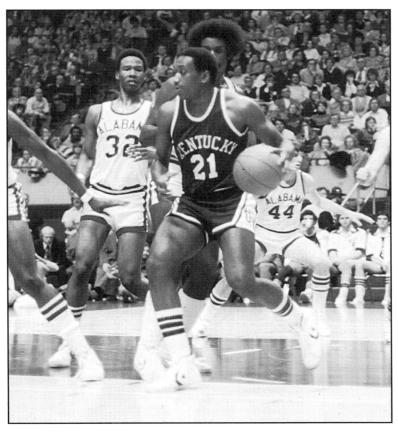

*Lexington native Jack "Goose" Givens could score in a number
of ways, which made him the main focus of opposing defenses.*

Kentucky's inside game which had been its strength with the seniors, Phillips, Robey, Givens and Lee, playing on the interior.
Michigan State's magnificent Earvin "Magic" Johnson was penetrat-
ing the UK defense and his clever passes set up his teammates for
easy baskets as the Spartans held the halftime lead, 27-22. Kentucky
had led early in the game, but Michigan State seemed to have
seized the momentum as the game went along.

In the UK dressing room, Hall pointed out to his team that
Michigan State had packed in the zone and closed down Ken-

tucky's inside game. He told them that Macy and Claytor would have to pick up the scoring from the outside. As the team went back out for the second half, Hamilton suggested to Hall that Kentucky use Robey to come out to the top of the key and set screens for Macy's jump shots. Hall bought his assistant's idea.

The team was already warming up for the second half when Hall yelled for Macy and Robey to come over to the UK bench. He told them the team would go to a 1-3-1 offense and that Robey would be setting the screens for Macy's outside shot. As Macy said, "It really worked." With a little more than six minutes to play, Robey set a perfect screen on Michigan State's Terry Donnelly just to the right side of the free throw circle. Macy connected and Donnelly fouled him. Macy cashed in the free throw and broke a 41-41 tie. The Cats were ahead to stay. Macy did not make another field goal, but as the Michigan State guards kept fighting through the screens, Macy kept going to the charity stripe. The Spartans tried to ice him on the line with two timeouts, but it failed to bother the 6-3 guard as he made six straight in the last three minutes and Kentucky won the Mideast Regional title, 52-49. Macy was named MVP for the regional. After the game, Robey underscored the versatility of that team when he said, "We proved we could do it anyway."

That team was a multi-faceted bunch. They could play fast-break teams or slow downs. They could adjust to about any style of play. "They were very unselfish," Hall noted. "In one game one player would be the hero and the next game it would be somebody else."

The four seniors had been freshmen at UK in 1975, when the Wildcats won the Mideast Regional in that same University of Dayton Arena. They told the underclassmen to expect a joyous celebration on the ride home down I-75. They were right in their prediction. Once the bus carrying the team crossed the Ohio River into Kentucky, a police escort led the journey to Lexington. All along the way, especially as the convoy traveled under bridges and overpasses, fans cheered, waved blue and white articles and held up homemade signs. I especially liked one that read "The Fabulous 14." That

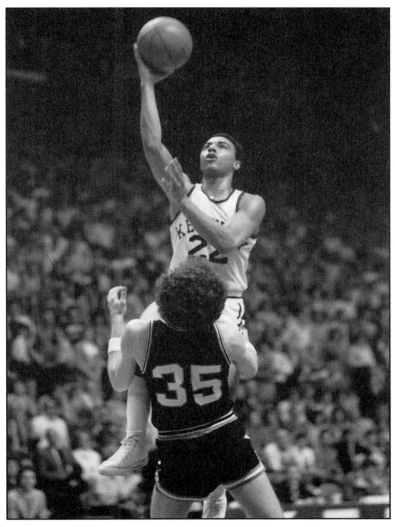

A lightning-quick guard, Truman Claytor was superb at turning great defensive plays into instant offense.

1978 group was really a team, one that involved all the players on the squad. At the end of the ride to Lexington, there was a wild reception in Memorial Coliseum.

Hall had seen all this in 1975 and he felt that his players never quite got over all the celebrating. They were beaten in the final game at San Diego. There, he had been completely accessible to the media. The players were permitted to go sightseeing. I know I enjoyed accompanying the team on their tour of the San Diego Zoo. Hall was determined that the trip to St. Louis for the 1978 Final Four would be a more serious trip.

Kentucky fans were out in force as the Wildcats went through their public practice in the Checkerdome on Friday. Kyle Macy noticed that the basket was too low and reported it to equipment manager Bill Keightley.

Kyle said, "Bill said Rick Robey had already complained about it." Keightley got it fixed.

Duke and Notre Dame opened the Final Four on Saturday afternoon with Duke's speed prevailing in the end, 90-86.

As Kentucky got ready to leave the dressing room to take on Arkansas, they heard all hell break loose in the Duke dressing room.

"You would have thought Duke had just won the championship," Hall was telling me recently. "They were yelling and hollering and I think they must have thrown Coach Bill Foster in the shower."

Hall had a lot of respect for the Arkansas team his Wildcats were facing. After the tournament was over and he was looking back, he said Arkansas might have been the best team his Wildcats faced all the way through the NCAA Tournament. The Razorbacks had three of the best players in the country in Sidney Moncrief, Marvin Delph and Ron Brewer, a trio of 6-4 guards. They called them the "Triplets."

"They all three were outstanding players," Hall said, "and Moncrief was just a super player."

The game was billed as Arkansas' quickness versus Kentucky's power. Kentucky's depth turned out to be an even bigger factor as fouls took their toll on a thinner Arkansas squad. Kentucky led most of the way but the Razorbacks kept fighting back. When the final horn sounded, the Cats were on top of what had been a brilliant basketball game, 64-59.

Throughout the season, Kentucky had been branded by some

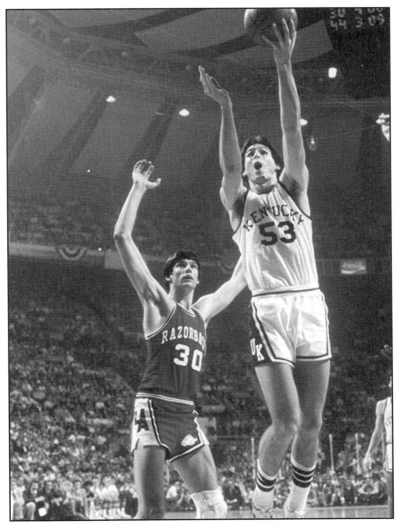

Rick Robey and the Cats held off a pesky Arkansas group in the semifinals of the 1978 NCAA Tournament.

coaches as taking the finesse out of the game. Perhaps with some jealousy showing, they had accused the Cats of brutalizing the game. True, Kentucky did have power with the 6-10 "Twin Towers" patrolling the inside, but Claytor and Givens, and to a lesser degree

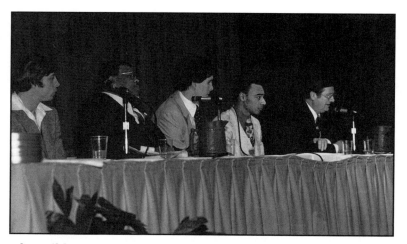

***The Wildcats were all business before the national title game
with Duke.***

Macy, brought some quickness to the team. Arkansas coach Eddie
Sutton, who was to be Hall's successor at Kentucky eight years
later, had high praise for the Wildcats. "Anybody who said Kentucky did not have quickness should have his head examined."

"That season was known as the year of no celebrating," recalled long-time UK equipment manager Bill Keightley. "I think
Joe B. really felt the pressure to win it that year. He had come
close but hadn't won it. Our fans were getting a little impatient
since it had been 20 years since the last championship."

After the Arkansas win, the players were whooping it up on the
way to the dressing room, but Keightley said Hall came through
and admonished the players, "No celebration. No celebration."

I was in the audience for the press conference on Sunday and
could tell from the tone of the questions to Hall that the stories
across the country the next day would be about the fun-loving
Duke youngsters going against the solemn, serious Kentucky players. When asked about that, Hall pulled no punches. "We're not
celebrating," he said. "We want to win the championship. We're
going to celebrate after it's over."

The lobby of Stouffer's Inn was packed morning, noon and night with fans dressed in blue. To get the players away from the hotel, Hall told Robey to get the players to choose a movie somewhere away from downtown. They would eat dinner near the theatre, then see a film.

"Robey asked me if we had taped the Duke-Notre Dame game," Hall said. "We had and he told me the players would rather stay in their rooms and watch the tape. We had it piped in their rooms and that's how they spent the evening before we went out to play for the national championship."

The next night Kentucky went out for their warmups before facing Duke. When the players returned to the dressing room and before they were joined by the coaches, the seniors called the team together just to remind everybody how close they were to reaching their goals. Those four seniors had provided great leadership to that team all season long.

When Hall came to the room, he walked to the blackboard and wrote the figure 40. That was to signify that the Cats were only 40 minutes away from the title. Then he went over the game plan. The biggest key, he told them, was to stop Duke's fast break. The Blue Devils had several runouts against Notre Dame for easy baskets. As Macy remembered, "I don't think they got a single one on us that night."

Duke was known for its stingy 2-3 zone defense. As Kentucky brought the ball over the center line, Hall noticed the Duke guards, the front two players in the zone, were picking up Kentucky's guards, Macy and Claytor, very far away from the basket. "I think they feared their outside shooting," Hall said. He also noticed that the three players along the base line were not coming out any. That left a big hole in the middle of the Duke zone.

"We had a pattern we called six-zone," Hall said. "We had run it for years. Coach Rupp had run it for a long time. The play had five or six options, depending on how the opponent played the zone. The first time we ran it, they didn't cover Givens when he

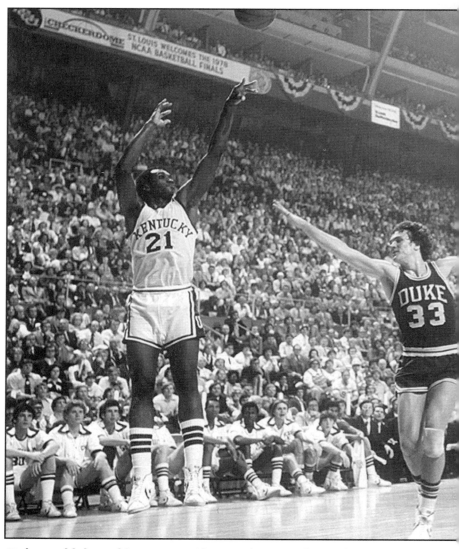

Duke could do nothing to stop Givens, who scored 41 points in being named the Most Outstanding Player of the Final Four.

flashed to the middle. During our timeout, I told our players to forget the other options. Just go to Jack's option."

Givens did the rest. Jack just shot the lights out. He not only

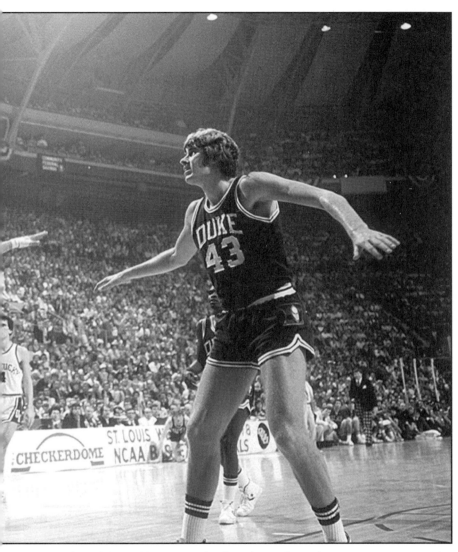

found himself open in the free throw lane, he was wearing out the net from everywhere. He scored 23 points in the first half to lead Kentucky to a 45-38 advantage at intermission. Jack didn't cool down any in the second half. From the left side of the floor he fired up a shot that hit the edge of the backboard and still went in the basket. "That's the kind of night I was having," Jack said. He was

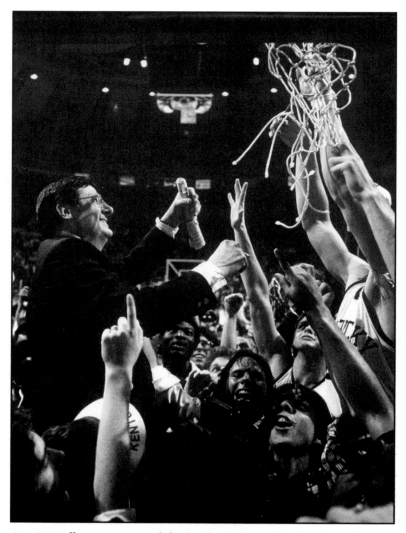

Joe B. Hall was on top of the basketball world after he guided UK to the 1978 national championship.

on his way to scoring 41 points in the game.

Givens was certainly the star of the show but it was not a one-man band. Robey had 20 points and 11 rebounds. Macy took only three shots but he hit them all. Kentucky led throughout the second half but when Hall put in the reserves with several minutes to go, Duke cut into the margin. The starters went back in and that was all she wrote. Lee supplied the perfect end to the game when he raced down court for one of his patented thunder dunks. Kentucky won, 94-88. Once again the blue and white banner of Kentucky was to fly over college basketball.

As the cheerleaders linked arms and joined the UK band for the singing of "My Old Kentucky Home," there was a feeling of joy and pride all over this Commonwealth ... a joy and pride Kentucky fans were experiencing for the first time in 20 years. This had been a season of no celebration, but now it was time for the celebration to begin.

The Best Team That Never Won the Title

If ever a college basketball team was well prepared for the approaching season, the 1953-54 Kentucky Wildcats had to be at the top of the list. Adolph Rupp had an entire season of practice to get them ready.

The University of Kentucky was one of seven schools implicated in the point-shaving scandal of the late 1940s, but the news broke several years later and the Wildcats were suspended from playing the entire 1952-53 season. First the Southeastern Conference voted to ban the Cats from competition, then the NCAA followed suit.

Rupp decided that he would approach the 1952-53 season just as if his team would be playing a schedule. They practiced every day and they practiced hard. The UK media guide lists four intrasquad games, but Gayle Rose, a member of that team, remembered two games against the Minneapolis Lakers before the start of the season. Rose recalled that the two teams split the games and in the game UK won, Cliff Hagan totally outplayed 6-10 George Mikan, one of the great pro stars of that day.

Rupp was especially driven. He had been implicated then cleared of the point-shaving charges, but he was angry about the whole deal and had vowed to "make those bastards pay." The

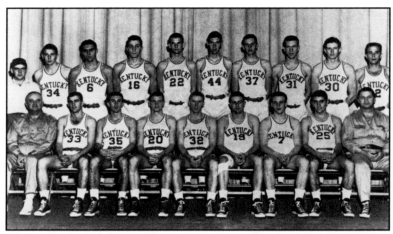

The 1953-54 Kentucky Wildcats. Front Row (L-R): Head Coach Adolph Rupp, Linville Puckett, Jess Curry, Gayle Rose, Clay Evans, Willie Rouse, Dan Chandler, Pete Grigsby, Asst. Coach Harry Lancaster. Back Row: Mgr. Mike Dolan, Hugh Coy, Cliff Hagan, Lou Tsioropoulos, Jerry Bird, Phil Grawemeyer, Harold Hurst, Bill Bibb, Frank Ramsey, Bill Evans.

1953-54 season was to be pay-back time.

That was the situation when I came on the scene in the early fall of 1953 to become the play-by-play announcer for the Wildcats. The furor had died down and everybody in the Commonwealth of Kentucky was excited about returning to competition after a 20-month absence.

Without question, Adolph Rupp was the king of college basketball in those days. He had already won three NCAA Championships, more than any other coach. I was absolutely in awe of the man as we met for the first time in his office. He couldn't have been more gracious. He took me on a tour of Memorial Coliseum and we had a great time. I was surprised that he would be so nice to a person he was meeting for the first time. I had heard all summer that he was so determined to demolish the opposition that he had installed an extra digit on the scoreboard so that he could run up the score. When I saw there were still only two digits on the board, I pointed it out to him. He had also heard the rumor and thought it was hilarious that I had brought it up. That was the beginning of our relationship that would last through his last 19 years as the coach at UK.

Kentucky was loaded with talent. Cliff Hagan, Frank Ramsey and Lou Tsioropoulos had been key players on the 1951 NCAA Championship team. The following year, Hagan and Ramsey were named to the All-American team. In Kentucky's storied basketball history, only three players have been enshrined in the Basketball Hall of Fame and two of those, Hagan and Ramsey, were on the 1953-54 team. It was several years later before Dan Issel joined the two.

Hagan was a scoring machine. He could shoot the hook shot with either hand and he could shoot it with accuracy 10 to 15 feet away from the basket. Cliff had an arsenal of shots. He was virtually unstoppable when he got the ball anywhere around the lane. If the opposition clogged the middle with a zone, Hagan was deadly accurate from the corner. Even through he was only 6-4, Rupp decided to play Cliff at center.

Ramsey was 6-3 and greased-lightning driving with the ball. He was tall for a guard in those days and if a smaller man was assigned to guard Frank, Ramsey would take him down inside and score effectively. Frank could play any position on the team and in one game, against Tennessee, he actually played center and turned in a great game. Ramsey could move, could shoot and could think. In a word, Frank Ramsey was a winner.

Lou Tsioropoulos was a superb athlete. He was also the only non-Kentuckian of the first seven players. Lou was 6-5 and was very strong. He had been an outstanding football player in high school in Lynn, Massachusetts. Tsioropoulos could score but it was his defense that made him invaluable to the Cats. Lou always took the other team's best inside player, whether he was a center or a forward.

Hagan, Ramsey and Tsioropoulos had been together their entire careers at Kentucky and, while sitting out of competition the prior year, all three had graduated and enrolled in graduate school. They referred to themselves as the "Big Three." They started every game the entire season. Billy Evans and Phil "Cookie" Grawemeyer shared

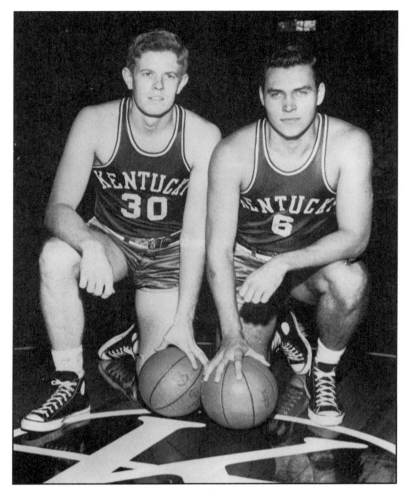

Frank Ramsey and Cliff Hagan, All-Americans during the 1953-54 season, are enshrined in the Basketball Hall of Fame.

the forward position opposite Tsioropoulos while Gayle Rose and Linville Puckett alternated at the guard position opposite Ramsey.

Starved for almost two years without basketball, the fans packed Memorial Coliseum as the Wildcats opened the season against Temple on December 5, 1953. That game will always be special to me. That was the first time I sat behind the microphone to provide play-by-play of the University of Kentucky.

The crowd was wild as the five Kentucky starters were introduced. Hagan, Ramsey and Tsioropoulos were joined by Evans and Rose for the opener against Temple. The Owls were expected to make a real game of it but it was all Kentucky right from the get-go. Hagan scored 20 points in the first half, the same total the entire Temple team had put on the scoreboard. Hagan scored 51 points to set a new UK and SEC scoring record. The Cats demolished Temple, 86-59.

Kentucky went on the road to win handily over Xavier then returned home to trounce Wake Forest. Then the Wildcats headed for St. Louis to take on their old nemesis, the St. Louis Billikens.

St. Louis seemed to have Kentucky's number. The last three meetings between the two teams had been in the Sugar Bowl Tournaments and the Billikens won all three — by a TOTAL of just four points. There was no love lost between Rupp and the St. Louis coach, Ed Hickey, and Rupp badly wanted to win the game.

The game was being played without incident but all hell was about to break loose on the sideline. Hickey's son was the timekeeper and at the end of each quarter (the college game was played in four 10-minute quarters in those days) young Hickey would fire a blank pistol to signal the end of the period. After the first quarter, he fired the pistol close to assistant coach Harry Lancaster and the wadding hit Harry on the leg. Lancaster said it was painful and he warned the young man about it. Lancaster told me that young Hickey told him to "go to hell." In Harry's further explanation of the incident, he recalled, "I informed him that if it occurred again, I was going to knock his ass off. Sure enough, as the half ended, he shot me again. I knocked his ass off."

A free-for-all followed but order was restored and the game continued. Lancaster won the fight and Kentucky won the game, 71-59. The undefeated Cats headed to Lexington to host the very first University of Kentucky Invitational Tournament.

Rupp and Bernie Shively, UK's Athletics Director, had generated the idea during the preceding year. They planned to invite four of

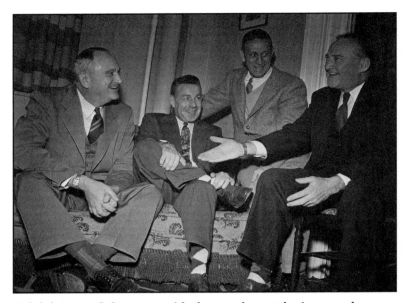

Adolph Rupp (left) meets with the coaches at the inaugural University of Kentucky Invitational Tournament. From left: Duke's Harold Bradley, UCLA's John Wooden and La Salle's Ken Loeffler.

the best teams from different parts of the country and bring them into Lexington during the Christmas break so that all the seats could be sold. After deducting expenses, the four teams would share equally in the proceeds. Duke, UCLA and La Salle joined Kentucky for the inaugural UKIT.

The Wildcats eliminated Duke the first night while La Salle measured UCLA. That set up the championship game. A great match was expected as La Salle had won the NIT the previous season and the Explorers featured one of the premier players of the game, Tom Gola.

The fans came to see a Hagan-Gola shootout. They came away singing the praises of both.

La Salle seized the momentum from the start. The Explorers raced out to a 13-4 lead. The starters for UK were small and La Salle was completely dominating the rebounding at both ends of the court. Rupp inserted 6-7 sophomore Phil Grawemeyer into the game, replacing the 6-0 Rose. Evans moved to guard and the Cats began to perk and by the end of the first quarter, they led, 16-13. At the half it was 32-29, in Kentucky's favor, and the Cats extended the lead to 45-38 by the end of the third quarter. Until that time, Tsioropoulos had held the talented Gola to only five points, but the La Salle star broke loose for 11 points in the fourth stanza. It was too little and too late as Kentucky won, 73-60.

Hagan had been magnificent in the battle of the two All-Americans, outscoring Gola, 23-16. Grawemeyer's entry into the game had been a shrewd move as he was outstanding on the boards as well as adding 13 points. Tsioropoulos, in addition to holding Gola to less than his average, actually outscored the La Salle star, 18-16.

The significance of the game would not be known until the end of the season. Kentucky declined an NCAA Tournament bid and La Salle went on to win the NCAA Championship.

Coach Rupp hadn't added the extra digit to the Coliseum scoreboard but he could have used it. Six times the Cats surpassed the century mark during the season and when they defeated Alabama at the end of the season, 68-43, they had a perfect 24-0 mark.

The Southeastern Conference was divided into three divisions in those days. Kentucky was grouped with Tennessee, Vanderbilt and Georgia Tech and they played twice each season. Kentucky played teams from the two other divisions just once each season, alternating between home and away.

The SEC ruled that for the 1953-54 season, the schedule would be the same as if Kentucky had played the year before. All the schools grudgingly agreed with the exception of LSU. The Tigers had an outstanding team that season, headed by the great Bob Pettit, and LSU was adamant that it would not travel to Lexington since Kentucky had skipped the trip to Baton Rouge, Louisiana, the year before. The teams did not play during the 1953-54 season and each went through the league undefeated. Bernie Moore, the SEC Commissioner at the time, ruled the two would meet at Vanderbilt's Memorial Gym in a playoff to determine the SEC Champion

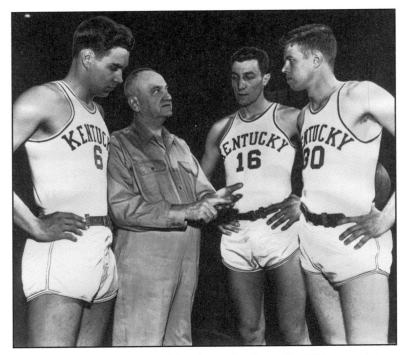

The 1953-54 team was led by the "Big Three," Cliff Hagan (6), Lou Tsioropoulos (16) and Frank Ramsey (30) with head coach Adolph Rupp.

and the league's representative in the NCAA Tournament.

Coach Rupp had suffered chest pains on the team's trip to Alabama at the end of the season and was ordered to bed the entire week prior to the game with LSU. He did accompany the team to Nashville the day before the game. On game day, March 9, 1954, Rupp suffered a mild heart attack and was under a doctor's care the entire day.

Lancaster accompanied the team from the Noel Hotel, in downtown Nashville, out to the arena on Vanderbilt's campus for the game. Just before the Wildcats left the bench for the start of the game, here came Rupp with Shively holding him steady by one arm. Coach Rupp was obviously ill but the man was tough as hickory. Leaning on Shively, Rupp gave his troops their last-minute instructions before they went out to face LSU.

Rupp, with Lancaster's help, had hatched his game plan earlier in the week. Kentucky's guards would pick up the LSU guards early in the half-court and keep pressure on them. Rupp's thinking was that it would help keep the ball away from Pettit. They knew UK would have to at least slow down the LSU star. Pettit had led the SEC in scoring for three years in a row. He was averaging more than 31 points and 17 rebounds a game going into the match with Kentucky. As usual, the very difficult defensive assignment went to Tsioropoulos.

The game lived up to expectations and was close all the way. When the final horn sounded, Kentucky had beaten the Bayou Bengals, 63-56.

Lancaster and Shively each took one of Rupp's elbows to escort him from the gym, but he insisted on visiting the Kentucky locker room first. The Cats had won the SEC Championship and the right to represent the conference in the NCAA Tournament.

I remembered that when Rupp was talking about Frank Ramsey earlier that season he had said, "If we win by 30, Frank will only get you three. If we win by three, he will get you 30." Well, Kentucky won by seven, but Ramsey led all scorers with 30 points. Hagan added 17 and Tsioropoulos held Pettit to 17, barely half his scoring average.

Back on January 25, 1954, Larry Boeck had written an article in *The Courier-Journal* that would change the destiny of that team. Boeck reported that Hagan, Ramsey and Tsioropoulos would not be eligible for the NCAA Tournament. They were all graduate students and under the rules they were eligible for the regular season but not for postseason play. Everybody seemed to be mad at Boeck but it was the UK front office who had goofed. If they had advised the three players to take fewer classes during the year they didn't play, they would have been eligible to play in the NCAA Tournament.

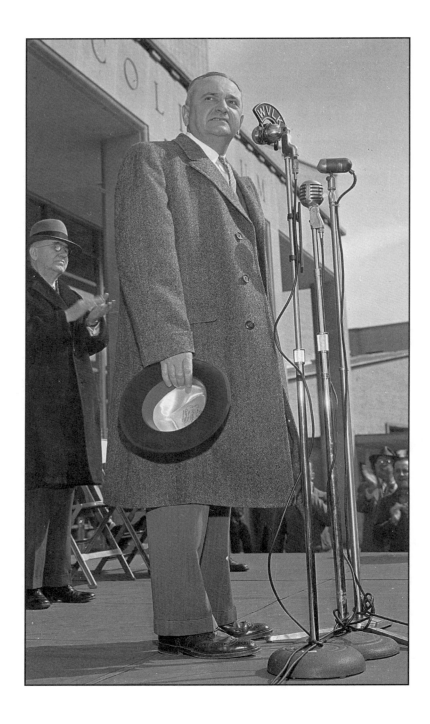

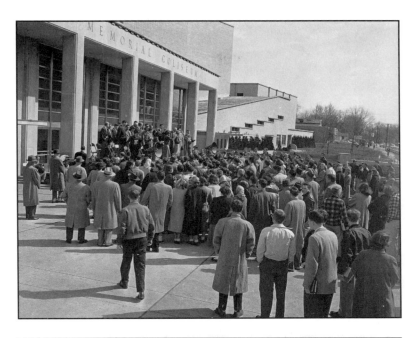

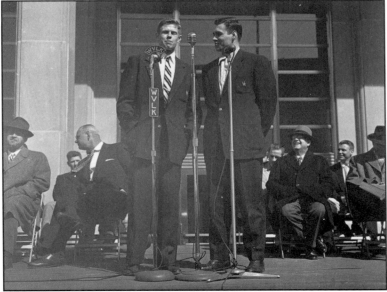

The Wildcats were met by throngs of Kentucky supporters after they completed the regular season at 24-0.

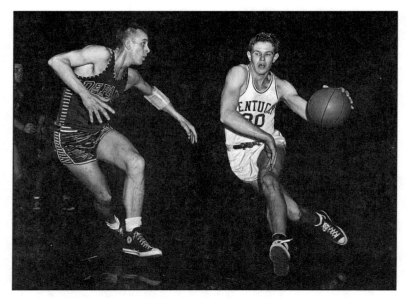

Frank Ramsey led Kentucky to victory with 30 points versus LSU in a playoff to determine the champion of the SEC.

Following the win over LSU, Rupp made his way to the dressing room and asked the players to vote on whether they wanted to go to the NCAA Tournament. Hagan, Ramsey and Tsioropoulos voted not to go, arguing that, without them, the team would have its perfect record marred. The players who were eligible all voted to go and the 9-3 vote meant the Cats were going to the NCAA Tournament. Coach Rupp never made much pretense at promoting a democracy in his program and he was to make the final decision this time, too. He told the team that since the three players had been the reason for a perfect season, UK would not go without them. He said, "I'm not going to take a bunch of turds like you to the NCAA." Case closed.

Gayle Rose remembered that while he was taking a shower, somebody came through to tell him that the jerseys of the top players would be retired. That took some of the sting out of not going to the tournament. Seven jerseys were retired — more than from any other UK team. The next time you're in Rupp Arena, look up to the rafters and you'll see the jerseys of Hagan, Ramsey, Tsioropoulos, Evans, Rose, Grawemeyer and Jerry Bird.

After the game, Shively assisted Rupp to a waiting taxi, and with a police escort, the pair made their way back to the hotel. After the three seniors had showered and dressed, they decided to visit their ailing coach. They found Rupp in his red pajamas and already in bed. When Hagan, Ramsey and Tsioropoulos asked him the secret of that team's great success, Rupp didn't miss a beat. "Hell, superior coaching," he said.

Kentucky stepped aside and allowed LSU to go to the NCAA Tournament but would always wonder what might have been. La Salle, a team the Wildcats had beaten by 13 points in the UKIT, won the national championship that year.

Still, that 25-0 Kentucky record was something to crow about. It was the only undefeated team Rupp had in his illustrious UK career.

In my mind, that 1953-54 Kentucky team was the best team that never won the NCAA Championship.

The Unbelievables

Lordy, that man can coach!

When Jim Host and I met in early January to discuss this book, no thought was given to including this chapter. Neither one of us could see Kentucky advancing very far in the NCAA Tournament. What the Cats did was go all the way to the final game before losing in overtime to Arizona.

Just when I think I've seen Rick Pitino turn in his best coaching efforts, he turns right around and does it one better. After I returned home from the 1997 Final Four, I sent Rick a note that read, "If there's ever been a better coaching job, I don't know about it." I said exactly what I meant. To take that team to the final game ... to be the 1997 runner-up in the NCAA Tournament, was truly a remarkable achievement.

Pitino faced a major rebuilding job for the 1996-97 season. From that marvelous team that won the NCAA Championship the previous season, four outstanding players departed. Antoine Walker, Tony Delk and Walter McCarty were drafted in the first round by NBA teams. Mark Pope went in the second round. With the three seniors departing and Walker leaving for the NBA after only two years, Kentucky lost its top three scorers, top three rebounders and most experienced players. Three starters, Walker, Delk and

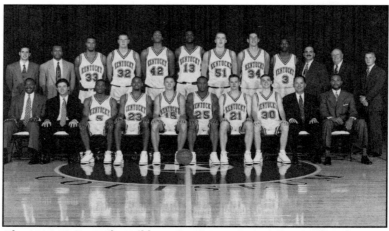

The 1996-97 Kentucky Wildcats. Front Row (L-R): Asst. Coach Delray Brooks, Head Coach Rick Pitino, Wayne Turner, Derek Anderson, Jeff Sheppard, Anthony Epps, Cameron Mills, Stephen Masiello, Assoc. Coach Jim O'Brien, Asst. Coach Winston Bennett. Back Row: Video Coord. Frank Vogel, Admin. Asst. Simeon Mars, Ron Mercer, Jared Prickett, Jamaal Magloire, Nazr Mohammed, Oliver Simmons, Scott Padgett, Allen Edwards, Trainer Eddie Jamiel, Equip. Mgr. Bill Keightley, Strength Coach Shaun Brown.

McCarty, plus an outstanding sixth man, Pope, were missing for the 1996-97 season.

Before the campaign got underway, I had a chance to talk with Pitino about the coming season. I told him it reminded me of the 1979 season. Kentucky had won the NCAA Championship in 1978, but lost three starters from that team: Rick Robey, Mike Phillips and Jack Givens. The best sixth man in the country, James Lee, departed as well. It was almost a carbon copy of what the Cats were losing going into the 1996-97 season. After winning the title in 1978, Kentucky posted a 16-10 record during the 1978-79 regular season. Those Cats did catch fire in the SEC Tournament, winning three games before losing in overtime to Tennessee in the final. They weren't chosen for the NCAA field, but had an NIT game in Rupp Arena, where they lost a second straight overtime decision. This time it was to Clemson as Kentucky finished the year with a record of 19-12.

I didn't think Kentucky would lose 12 games, but I thought the 1996-97 season could be a rocky ride. Rick felt it would be especially difficult early with a tough schedule away from friendly Rupp Arena, but he thought by March the Wildcats could be in the hunt to defend their national title. I admired his optimism.

Kentucky had its earliest opening game in history when the Cats headed to Indianapolis for the Black Coaches' Association Classic against the veteran Clemson Tigers on November 15. Clemson had all five starters returning from the prior season.

The Wildcats had two starters back from the championship team, Anthony Epps and Derek Anderson. Epps had been the starting point guard while Anderson had been in the opening lineup at the small forward position. Pitino switched him to Tony Delk's two-guard spot, thinking it was the natural position for Anderson. Epps would not make the starting lineup, as Pitino had decided on sophomore Wayne Turner to run the UK offense.

Jared Prickett started at center in the opening game. The 6-9, 235-pound senior had played in only five games the previous season. He was not fully recovered from a wounded knee and had received a medical hardship ruling. Prickett brought a lot of hustle and moxy to the team and with McCarty, Pope and Walker gone from the inside, the Cats welcomed Jared back.

Ron Mercer and Allen Edwards were the starting forwards against Clemson. This gave the Cats a pony-sized frontcourt. Edwards, a 6-5, 205-pound junior, was considered a swing player, alternating between the two-guard position and the small forward. Pitino felt that Edwards was the most versatile player on the team and that he really understood the game. He had started only one game during his first two seasons at UK.

Mercer, a 6-7, 210-pound sophomore, came out of high school ranked as the best player in the country. He started the first dozen games as a freshman before going to the bench to be brought along more slowly. He was fifth in scoring that year and ended the season with a bang, scoring 20 points in the NCAA final. He was no secret and was named to the preseason All-SEC team.

Kentucky certainly lacked the depth it had enjoyed the preceding year. Pitino could call on Epps, who had great experience, but after that it was a green bunch who sat with him on the bench. Cameron Mills had just been put on scholarship after playing as a walk-on for two years. Both he and sophomore Nazr Mohammed had seen most of their action with the junior varsity team. Jamaal Magloire was an incoming freshman and Oliver Simmons was a sophomore who had not seen a lot of action. Oliver, too, had seen most of his duty with the junior varsity team. He would play briefly in the opening game, then decide to transfer to Florida State.

The season began for the Cats in the RCA Dome in Indianapolis, and the Kentucky players were hoping that they would return there at the end of the campaign. The RCA Dome was to be the site of the Final Four.

Kentucky got off to a good start against the Tigers and led at the half, 37-31. Midway through the second half, Clemson began to gain momentum and when the buzzer sounded, the two teams were deadlocked, 63-63. Clemson's inside players dominated in overtime and the Tigers clawed out a 79-71 decision.

Pitino realized that his small lineup had suffered at the hands of the bigger Clemson players. The Cats had trouble defensively against the bulkier Tigers and Clemson had pummeled UK on the boards, outrebounding the Cats, 44-28. He would change that when the Cats next took the court in the Great Alaska Shootout.

Prickett, at 6-9, would move from center to replace Edwards at a forward position. Mohammed moved into the pivot and Pitino decided that Epps would again start at the point instead of Turner.

Mohammed brought size to the center position. The 6-10 sophomore had lost more than 60 pounds since coming to UK and now he checked in at a svelte 238 pounds.

Before the season began, Pitino had said of Epps, "Next to the definition of winner in Webster's Dictionary should be Anthony's picture." Epps was promoted and demoted throughout his career at

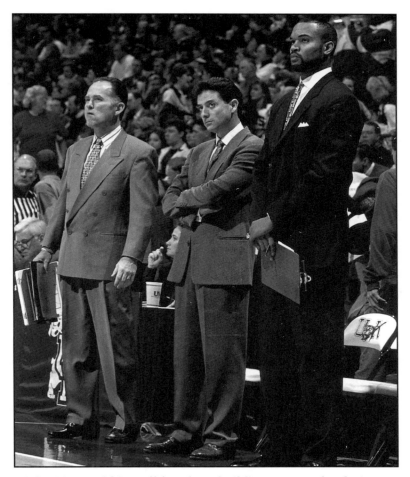

Rick Pitino and his staff faced a rebuilding season after losing three starters and a number of contributors from the 1996 national championship team. Here, Pitino is flanked by assistant coaches Jim O'Brien (left) and Winston Bennett (right).

UK, but to his everlasting credit, he took both in stride. Each time he lost his starting position, and it was fairly frequent, Anthony just rolled up his sleeves, spit on his hands and went to work. There was never any pouting or whining and now he was back in the starting lineup.

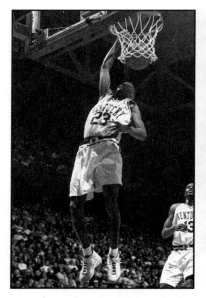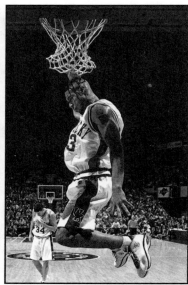

Derek Anderson (left) and Ron Mercer (right), the self-dubbed "Air Pair," were a lethal combination for opponents.

As the action began in Anchorage, Alaska, Kentucky found it-self in a contest with Syracuse, the team the Cats defeated in the NCAA championship game for the 1996 national title. It was no contest as the Wildcats handed coach Jim Boeheim the worst loss of his career, 87-53. Pitino got the big game out of his 6-10 cen-ter, but it wasn't Mohammed, it was Jamaal Magloire. The big freshman came off the bench to score 16 points, grab eight re-bounds and would move into the starting lineup for the next game. The two 6-10 centers would become interchangeable for the remainder of the season.

Kentucky breezed to the Great Alaska Shootout title by dispatch-ing Alaska-Anchorage and the College of Charleston in easy fashion.

UK completed its 10,000 mile journey by stopping off in Chica-go and defeating Purdue in the Great Eight.

The Cats faced Indiana in Louisville's Freedom Hall and hand-ed Bob Knight one of the worst losses in his storied career as the

Cats exploded for a 99-65 win. Anderson and Mercer were becoming one of the most lethal one-two punches in the college game. Anderson scored 30 points and Mercer 26 in the win over the Hoosiers.

Pitino's road warriors played seven of their first nine games away from Rupp Arena. The ninth game was significant because Kentucky, for a change, was going to gain a player. After an 18-month absence, Scott Padgett rejoined the Cats. When Padgett accompanied the Wildcats to Italy, he knew he would not be eligible the following season because of academic shortcomings. Scott had played well in Italy, leading the Cats in three-point accuracy. Even though he had been on the UK team for a year, it was the first time Pitino saw just how good he was. "Scott Padgett really came into his own in Italy and we knew we would have a good player down the road, if he got his act straightened out," Pitino said.

Scott got his act together. He really buckled down on the books and made the dean's list. He became eligible to rejoin the team as Kentucky headed to Atlanta to meet Georgia Tech on December 21, 1996. The twin scorers, Anderson and Mercer, led the parade with 21 and 20 points, respectively, as Kentucky overpowered Tech, 88-59. Padgett made quite a debut, coming off the bench to score 12 points and grab seven rebounds.

Three games later, Kentucky returned to Freedom Hall for its annual game against the Louisville Cardinals. Pitino elevated Padgett into the starting lineup, replacing Prickett at forward. Scott scored 15 points and with another Louisvillian, Derek Anderson, leading five UK players in double figures with 19, the Cats broke open a close game in the second half and rolled to a 74-54 win.

Kentucky had posted a 14-game winning streak, which included a 2-0 start in the SEC race, when the Cats made their first conference road trip to Oxford, Mississippi, on January 11. Anderson had a pulled back muscle and failed to start against Ole Miss. He saw only five minutes of action, but was far below par and went

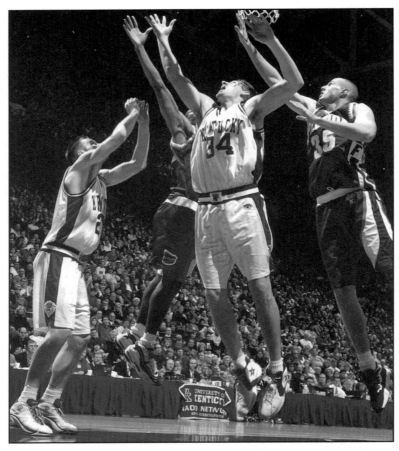

***Scott Padgett's return to UK gave the Wildcats a much-needed
boost in the frontcourt.***

scoreless for the first time all season. The hot-shooting Ole Miss
Rebels upset the Cats, 73-69. The Cats rebounded against Georgia,
in Athens, as Anderson returned to the lineup and led UK in scoring with 24 points.

Back in Rupp Arena, Kentucky breezed past Auburn, 77-53, but
it was a bittersweet victory. Rick Pitino won his 200th game as the
UK coach, but Anderson went down in the second half with what
was thought to be a bruised knee. The injury proved much more

serious. He later had to undergo surgery and was lost to the Wildcats for the remainder of the season.

In my opinion, Anderson was the best player on the Kentucky
roster. The 6-5 senior was leading Kentucky and the Southeastern
Conference in scoring. Derek had blazing speed, quickness and
great jumping ability. He was explosive at both ends of the court
and now any hopes Kentucky had in postseason play had surely
gone down the drain with Anderson's injury.

Pitino, as usual, embraced the challenge. He told his players
that each one of them would have to improve his performance by
20 percent.

Edwards moved into Anderson's spot and while the Cats struggled a bit for a few games, they were winning. Kentucky had lost
only one conference game as it headed to Columbia, South Carolina, to play the Gamecocks. South Carolina was undefeated in
league play, so this was a major confrontation in the SEC. Prickett
had injured his ankle the day before and would not play, leaving
Pitino with only eight scholarship players available. It was a hard-
fought game that saw one team, then the other, go on scoring
binges. With 1:25 left in the game, Edwards' jumpshot gave Kentucky a 74-69 lead and the Cats appeared to be in great shape.
Some sloppy UK ball-handling and five straight points from Carolina tied the game and sent it into overtime. The Gamecocks went
on to win, 84-79. UK had now lost two conference games while
South Carolina was undefeated in league play. It was going to be
an uphill battle for Kentucky.

The resilient Cats once again made a comeback, running off
seven straight wins. The most exciting game in that string and perhaps the most exciting game of the season came when Kentucky
visited Vanderbilt's Memorial Gymnasium in Nashville.

Kentucky usually has trouble in Music City and this game was
no exception. After the score was tied at seven early, the Com-
modores went on a scoring spree. Vandy was on top by 22 with
3:51 remaining in the first half, 40-18. Just when it appeared it was

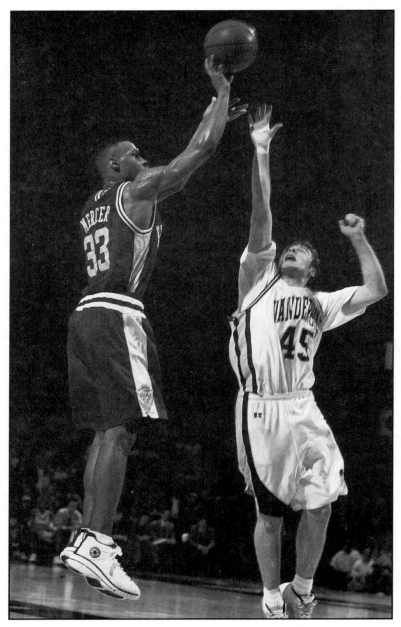

In his hometown of Nashville, Ron Mercer led the Cats back from a big deficit.

going to be a Vanderbilt romp, the Cats fought back. Turner hit his only three-point shot of the game just as the horn halted play in the first half and Kentucky had cut its deficit to 10, 44-34. Nashville native Mercer, playing in his hometown, scored 17 of his game-high 23 points in the second half as Kentucky completed its remarkable comeback to win, 82-79.

The regular season came to an end in Rupp Arena on March 2, as Kentucky entertained South Carolina. The Gamecocks had lost at Georgia, but still led the East Division with a 14-1 league record. Kentucky was in second place with a 13-2 worksheet. A Wildcat win would no doubt extract some measure of revenge for that earlier loss to Carolina, but it would also elevate the Cats into a tie for the division title. Under the tie-breaking system used by the SEC, Kentucky would be the top seed for the conference tournament.

As if the game needed any extra hype, this was Senior Day, the time set aside each season for the fans to say farewell to those seniors who have meant so much to the UK basketball program. Anderson, Epps and Prickett ran through hoops bearing their likeness before the game, the band played "My Old Kentucky Home," and the 24,326 fans in Rupp Arena were at a frenzy as the opening tip-off rolled around.

South Carolina's three quick guards, Melvin Watson, Larry Davis, and BJ McKie, slashed into the Kentucky defense, either scoring or, more often, drawing fouls. The Gamecocks shot 44 free throws to Kentucky's 15 and won another close battle from the Cats, 72-66. Pitino was banished from the game with four-tenths of a second left after picking up two technical fouls. He later apologized for his actions.

Pitino was not a happy camper after watching the videotape of the game. With the SEC Tournament just days away, he announced that Prickett would replace Magloire at center and Turner would take over the point guard position from Epps. Pitino figured Prickett would be more effective on the press and would make Kentucky a better passing team. He thought Turner would give them more quickness on both offense and defense.

The regular season was over. Kentucky led in most of the SEC statistical categories, but had to settle for second place in the league standings. Ron Mercer reaped the postseason awards. He was on the first-team All-SEC, Player of the Year in the conference and a first-team All-American.

The Wildcats headed for Memphis and the SEC Tournament. Auburn defeated Tennessee on Thursday and would be the Wildcats' opponent the following day. Prickett intercepted the opening tip-off and threw a lob to Mercer for a dunk and the Cats were off and running with a 2-0 lead. They never looked back and breezed to an easy 92-50 win.

If Kentucky hadn't embraced bad luck, it would have had no luck at all. Edwards was nursing a bad back, an injury suffered in practice. He played only five minutes and told Pitino he couldn't go. The Cats had been plagued with one setback after another all season long and now they would likely be going the rest of the way without Allen.

Next up for the Cats was Ole Miss, the first conference team to defeat Kentucky that season and the champion of the Western Division.

Pitino started Edwards but the junior forward didn't fire and left the game in only two minutes. If that Kentucky team was anything, it was resilient. Another understudy was ready to step from the wings onto center stage. This time it was Mills. The former walk-on came off the bench to score a career-high 14 points, including 4 of 6 from three-point range. Epps came off the bench to score 18 and Mercer was Mercer, stepping up like the All-American he was to lead the Wildcats with 19. It was an easy 88-70 win over Ole Miss.

Kentucky thought it would be meeting South Carolina in the final but Georgia knocked off the Gamecocks in the other semifinal and the Bulldogs would face Kentucky for the title.

Kentucky's up-tempo offense and pressure defense took Georgia out of the game early and the Cats had one of their easiest wins,

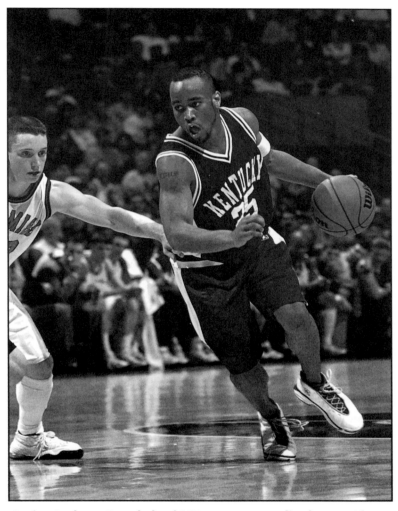

Senior Anthony Epps helped UK avenge an earlier loss to Ole Miss with a SEC Tournament semifinal victory.

95-68. With the injury to Edwards, Epps moved back into the starting position, but instead of his regular point guard position, Anthony played the two-guard. He led the Cats with 22 points. Mills continued his hot shooting with 16 points and Edwards, who was not expected to play, came into the game and scored 12 points,

163

two of which were sure to make the highlight film. Allen drove the baseline and just as he was confronted by two Georgia defenders, rose from the floor and threw home a wondrous dunk.

The star-crossed junior later came out with a gimpy ankle. It was first diagnosed as a sprain, but it would turn out to be much more serious — a stress fracture to the right foot.

Kentucky won the SEC Tournament for the 20th time and for the fifth time in the past six years. Mercer was named the tournament's MVP. Prickett, who earned a starting berth just before the tournament started, was named to the All-Tournament team. Epps, who lost his starting job at the same time Prickett was promoted, also made the All-Tournament team. Pitino was euphoric over the way his team played throughout the three-game shootout. "Since I've been here, we have not played three games as well offensively and defensively, from an execution standpoint."

After the game, Pitino was pleased to learn that his team would be a No. 1 seed in the NCAA Tournament. He was not pleased the Cats would be sent far from home to play in the West Region.

On March 13, Kentucky found itself 1,765 miles from home at the Huntsman Center in Salt Lake City, Utah, to begin the defense of its title. A No. 1 seed has never lost to a No. 16 seed in the tournament and Kentucky did not want to be the first. That's the situation UK faced as it met the Montana Grizzlies. The two teams fussed around for the first 10 minutes but Kentucky began to pull away and went on to an easy win, 92-54. Turner was really taking to his new starting role and cashed in with 19 points. Mills was again magnificent coming off the bench with another career-high 19.

Pitino was noticeably worried about the next opponent, Iowa. He called Iowa the best eight seed he had ever seen in the tournament and the Hawkeyes were going to make him a prophet.

With Mercer and Turner in early foul trouble, Prickett and Mills were left to carry the scoring load in the first half. Prickett tallied 15 points and Mills added 11, including three three-pointers, but the Cats could do no better than break-even and the two teams

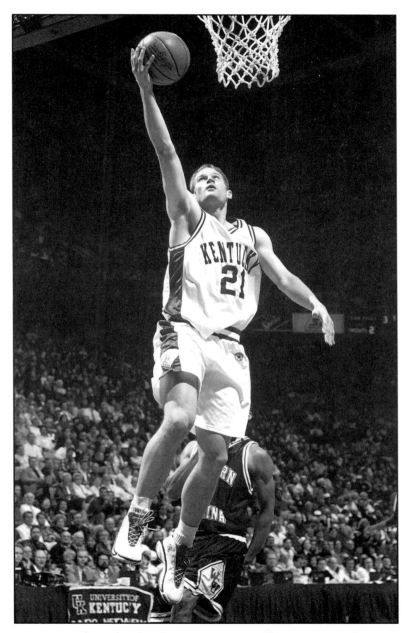

Unexpected production from Cameron Mills gave Kentucky's offense a new dimension late in the season.

were deadlocked at the intermission, 35-35.

This one went right down to the wire. With just 49 seconds left, Kentucky was clinging to a 72-69 lead after Iowa's magnificent guard, Andre Woolridge, drained a three-pointer. Padgett's 10-footer sealed it for the Cats as they gutted out a tough 75-69 win.

It was obvious this rag-tag group of Cats had gotten to the coach. After the game Pitino said, "I just love them to death."

The Wildcats had joined the Sweet 16 of college basketball and their reward was to just keep moving west ... another 765 miles west to San Jose, California.

First up, St. Joseph's, a team noted for firing an abundance of three-pointers — 30 or more a game. The UK defense held them to three treys out of only nine attempts and the Cats coasted to an 83-68 victory.

The Kentucky contingent held its breath during the game when Padgett went to the floor and was in obvious pain. With Anderson and Edwards already out, it could have been a disaster. But after a short stay on the bench, Padgett came back into the game and everyone breathed a sigh of relief. "When they said he could go back in the game, I was thankful," Pitino said. "Very thankful."

The top-seeded Wildcats would meet Utah, the No. 2 seed in the West Region final for the right to advance to the Final Four. Kentucky had beaten Utah 101-70 in the regional semifinals the preceding year, but to talk of a rematch from one year to another is usually an error in college basketball. Kentucky had only one starter from the 1996 team and Epps was starting at a different position.

The game was billed as a duel between two All-Americans, Kentucky's Mercer and Utah's Keith Van Horn. Mercer won that battle, outscoring Van Horn 21-15. Winning the game was more difficult.

Before the game, Pitino had predicted that Utah would eliminate the sensational scoring run Mills had enjoyed through the SEC and NCAA Tournaments. Mills was a spot-up shooter and his prowess from behind the three-point line would not be ignored by the Utah coaching staff. Mills was shut out for the only time in the tournament.

The contest developed into a roller coaster game with first one team then the other going in spurts. A run by the Utes in the second half tied the score at 43 with 9:40 remaining. Pitino called a timeout.

Mercer was brilliant in the first half with 15 points but he hadn't scored in the second half. With his players gathered around him on the sideline, Pitino told Mercer he would have to step up like the All-American he was if Kentucky was going to win. Then he took his coaching board and drew a line down the middle. On one side he wrote the word "winner," on the other side he wrote the word "loser." He told them they could leave the huddle a winner or a loser. He told them, "It's your choice."

It took Mercer only 17 seconds to respond as he hit a jumper from the baseline. He added another basket shortly after to push the Cats to a four-point lead. The other players caught the fever and the Wildcats sprinted away, winning over Utah, 72-59.

Kentucky had won the West Region Championship and would join the other three regional winners in Indianapolis for the Final Four. It was the second straight year for the Wildcats to reach the charmed circle.

All the Kentucky players had made a great contribution in the NCAA Tournament. Mercer was named MVP of the West Region and Wayne Turner joined him on the All-Tournament team. Even Anderson got into the action but it won't show in the record books. As Kentucky was killing the clock near the end of the game with six seconds to the final horn, Anderson sprinted from the bench on his rebuilt knees. Pitino didn't know it. The officials ignored it. Anderson gave Epps a big bear hug and the game was over.

Pitino was still sticking by his decision not to play Anderson at the Final Four but thought Edwards would be able to see spot duty in Indianapolis.

Rick Pitino shared in the ceremonial cutting down of the nets then expressed the feeling of most Kentucky fans when he said, "Now the fun starts!"

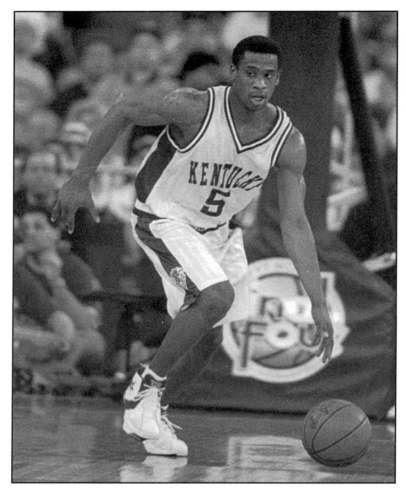

Rick Pitino made a key postseason adjustment by shifting Wayne Turner to point guard and Anthony Epps to shooting guard.

Frances and I drove to Indianapolis as guests of our long-time friends, Jim and Pat Host on Thursday, March 27, for the Final Four Salute Presentation honoring the four coaches. Lou Rawls was scheduled for a special appearance. I enjoyed spending some time with Clem Haskins, who would be coaching Minnesota against Kentucky on Saturday. Clem is an old friend who had been a spectacular player at Western Kentucky and had fashioned a fine coaching record with the Hilltoppers.

I stopped by Rick's table and he invited me to join the team the next morning for its private practice.

The NCAA mandates that each team at the Final Four hold a one-hour public practice on Friday, but in reality, those are just for show. All the teams have a private practice at some other gym. Obviously, none of them want the prying eyes of enemy scouts in the stands.

On Friday morning, Ralph Beard and I caught a cab to Kentucky's hotel. Ralph had been a three-time All-American at UK in the '40s and saw a brilliant, but brief, pro career snuffed out when he was involved in the point-shaving scandal. As the years have gone by, Ralph is less reluctant to talk about his problems and has been speaking to teams about the dangers of gambling. He had spoken to the NCAA Basketball Committee the day before and some of them told me he had given a great talk.

Ralph and I sat in as Associate Coach Jim O'Brien held a video session with the players. I've seen many of those sessions over the years but I'm still amazed at how meticulous and exacting these Kentucky encounters are. It's little wonder how well prepared the Wildcats are on the playing floor.

We rode the team bus to Warren Central High School's gym where Pitino put the Cats through their private practice session. They looked sharp. Anderson took shooting drills with the team but was held out of practice. As I watched, I couldn't help playing "what if?" What if Jeff Sheppard had not been redshirted? He looked terrific in practice and could really help the short-handed Wildcats. Before the season began, Pitino had decided to redshirt the 6-3 guard because he would be playing behind the talented Anderson and would have limited playing time. Rick thought Sheppard had the skills to have an opportunity to make it to the NBA and he would get the chance to show those skills after Anderson played out his eligibility. I thought Rick might reconsider the status

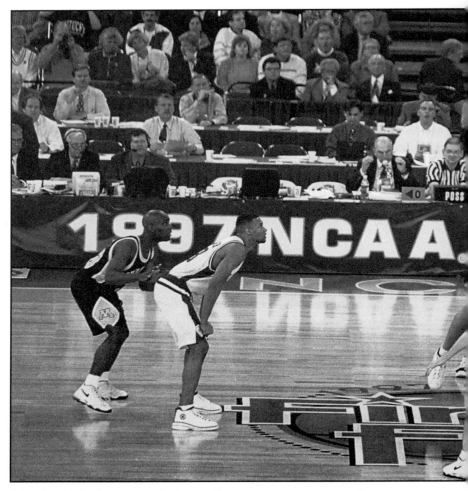

The 1997 Final Four marked UK's first repeat appearance since its Golden Era.

of Sheppard after Anderson was injured and lost for the season but he never wavered in his decision. He felt it would be unfair to Jeff for him to give up half of the season.

For only the second time in history, three top-seeded teams, Kentucky, Minnesota and North Carolina, made it to the Final Four. Arizona was the upstart, seeded only fourth in the Southeast, but

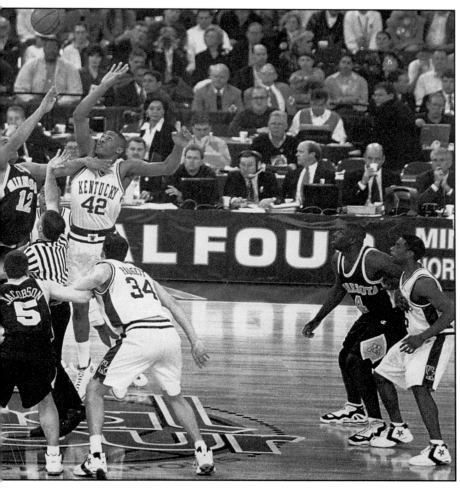

Lute Olson's Wildcats had upset top-seeded Kansas. The Jayhawks had been favored, not only to win the Southeast Region, but to win the entire tournament.

Arizona and North Carolina opened the 1997 Final Four. Carolina's Dean Smith had broken Adolph Rupp's record during the NCAA Tournament and came to Indianapolis with 879 wins, the most of any coach in college basketball history. Smith could also point to two NCAA Championships in his 36 years as the coach at North Carolina. Olson was still looking for his first NCAA title. Carolina was a five-point favorite and looked the part in the early going, racing to an 11-point lead. But Arizona caught up and actually moved ahead by the end of the first half, 34-31. Arizona was in control throughout the second half and upset the Tar Heels, 66-58. Arizona's pair of guards, Miles Simon and Mike Bibby, combined for 44 points to wreck Carolina.

Kentucky was more than a six-point favorite over Minnesota in the other semifinal game. The Cats had Edwards back, at least for spot duty, to give them more depth again. Pitino had studied the Golden Gophers and knew his Wildcats were in for a tough game against the Big Ten champions.

Kentucky got off to a quick start and when, early in the game, Mercer turned in one of his spectacular 360-degree spins for a layup, the 47,028 fans could feel the excitement. Unfortunately, Mercer's touch left him and he and his teammates struggled offensively through the first half. Kentucky's suffocating pressure defense held Minnesota at bay and the Cats led at halftime, 36-31.

The second half was even more bizarre. Mercer suffered leg cramps and sat out much of the half but still led Kentucky in scoring with 19. Haskins was tagged with a technical and Pitino sent Anderson, who hadn't played in more than two months, in to shoot the two free throws. He made both, then went back to the safety of the Kentucky bench. Minnesota took its only lead at 52-51 but again Kentucky was up to the challenge and hung on to win, 78-69.

The Kentucky defense had done it again. The Gophers coughed up the ball 26 times, 12 more than their season average. "We were scared," said Big Ten Player of the Year Bobby Jackson.

Kentucky was headed for a championship showdown with Arizona.

Kentucky was trying to win the title for the second straight year. Arizona was trying to win the school's first NCAA Championship.

The two teams went at it toe-to-toe right from the outset. In the first half alone, the score was tied on eight occasions and the lead changed hands 10 times before Arizona edged ahead at the inter-

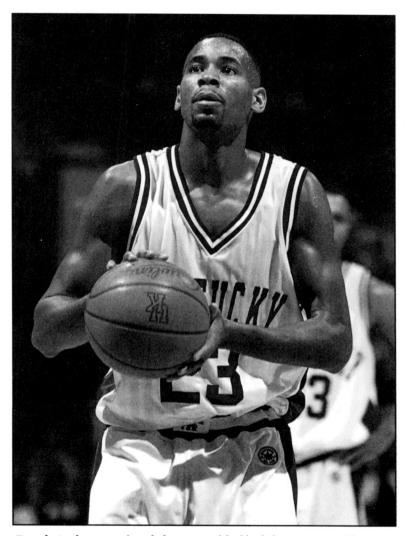

Derek Anderson missed the second half of the season with a knee injury, but he gave the Cats a boost by converting two technical free throws against Minnesota.

mission, 33-32.

The second half was a replay of the first. Near the end, it appeared that Arizona had pulled it out, leading by three. Anthony

Epps connected from behind the arc to tie the score and to send the game into overtime.

Arizona outscored Kentucky 10-5 in the extra period with all of Arizona's points coming at the free throw line. Kentucky committed 29 personal fouls and Mercer, Prickett, Turner and Padgett fouled out. Still, there were 15 ties and 19 lead changes before Arizona prevailed, 84-79.

Kentucky had fought its guts out but came up short. Barely. Rick Pitino told his charges that they had shown such heart and character they should feel like champions.

Pitino called them the "Unbelievables." They were.

"God, I am so proud of these guys," Rick proclaimed.

To that, we all say "Amen!"